Aids to Radiological Differential Diagnosis

Aids to Radiological Differential Diagnosis

Stephen Chapman

MB, BS, MRCP, FRCR

Department of Radiology
Birmingham Children's Hospital;
Senior Clinical Lecturer
University of Birmingham;
Formerly Tutor in Radiodiagnosis
University of Bristol

Richard Nakielny

MA, BM, BCh, FRCR

Department of Radiodiagnosis
Bristol Royal Infirmary;
Tutor in Radiodiagnosis
University of Bristol

Baillière Tindall London Philadelphia Toronto
Sydney Tokyo

| Baillière Tindall | 24–28 Oval Road |
| W. B. Saunders | London NW1 7DX |

West Washington Square
Philadelphia, PA 19105, USA

1 Goldthorne Avenue
Toronto, Ontario M8Z 5T9, Canada

ABP Australia Ltd, 44–50 Waterloo Road
North Ryde, NSW 2113, Australia

Harcourt Brace Jovanovich Japan Inc
Ichibancho Central Building, 22 -1 Ichibancho
Chiyoda-ku, Tokyo 102, Japan

© 1984 Baillière Tindall

First published 1984
  Reprinted 1985, 1986 (twice), 1988

Typeset by Activity Ltd, Salisbury
Printed and bound in Great Britain by
William Clowes Ltd, Beccles and London

British Library Cataloguing in Publication Data

Chapman, Stephen, *1953 –*
  Aids to radiological differential diagnosis.
  1. Diagnosis, Radioscopic
  I. Title   II. Nakielny, Richard
  616.07'57   RC78

ISBN 0-7020-1043-X

Contents

PART 2

Foreword

It is axiomatic that the single most important feature of managing an illness is making the diagnosis and that the first condition for making the diagnosis is to have in mind the possibility of its presence. Hence the popularity of exhaustive lists of causes of various radiological syndromes. One of the major difficulties encountered by candidates preparing for higher qualifications is acquiring the skill to reduce an exhaustive list to a short list of diagnostic probabilities in their correct order. Their inability to do so is often a disappointment for their examiners. Drs Chapman and Nakielny have written a text that will help the inexperienced through that very taxing period after they have become familiar with the fundamental concepts of radiodiagnosis and need a logical guide to their application.

There is no substitute for experience, but hastening its acquisition and helping to broaden its scope will no doubt be the main rewards for those who wish to benefit from the authors' diligent compilation.

E. Rhys Davies

Preface

During the period of study prior to taking the final Fellowship of the Royal College of Radiologists, or other similar radiological examinations, many specialist textbooks and the wealth of radiological papers are carefully scoured for lists of differential diagnoses of radiological signs. These will supplement the information already learned and enable that information to be used logically when analysing a radiograph. All this takes precious time when effort is best spent trying to memorize these lists rather than trying to find them within the massive texts or, even worse, trying to construct them oneself.

Consequently we decided to write a book which contains as many useful lists as one might reasonably be expected to know for a postgraduate examination. To make it manageable we have omitted those lists and conditions which have limited relevance to routine radiological practice. In addition, many of the lists are constructed in terms of a 'surgical sieve' and by using this method we would hope that the lists are easier to remember. We have tried to present the conditions in some order of importance, although we realize that local patient selection and the geographical distribution of diseases will have a great influence in modifying the lists. The lists will, almost certainly, not be acceptable to all radiologists. However, the basic lists are supplemented with useful facts and discriminating features about each condition and these should enable the trainee to give a considered opinion of the radiograph. So that this added information can be kept concise and to avoid unnecessary repetition we have summarized the radiological signs of many important conditions separately in Part 2 of the book.

The book has no radiographs. We have assumed a basic knowledge of radiology in the reader and expect him or her to already be able to recognize the abnormal signs. A limited number of line drawings have been used to emphasize radiographic abnormalities.

The aim of the book is to assist with logical interpretation of the radiograph. It is not intended for use on its own because it is not a complete radiological textbook. Recourse will need to be made to the larger general and specialist texts and journals and the reading of them is still a prerequisite to passing the postgraduate examinations.

More exhaustive lists are to be found in Felson & Reeder's *Gamuts in Radiology* (Pergamon Press, Oxford, 1975) and Kreel's *Outline of Radiology* (Heinemann, London, 1971) and these books are to be commended.

Stephen Chapman
Richard Nakielny

Explanatory Notes

The 'surgical sieve' classification used in the longer lists is presented in order of commonness, e.g. when 'neoplastic' is listed first then this is the commonest cause as a group. Within the group of neoplastic conditions, number 1 is more common or as common as number 2. However, it does not necessarily follow that all the conditions in the first group are more common than those in subsequent groups, e.g. infective, metabolic, etc.

The groups entitled 'idiopathic' or 'others' are usually listed last even though the disease or diseases within them may be common. This has been done for the sake of neatness only.

In order that the supplementary notes are not unnecessarily repeated in several lists, those conditions which appear in several lists are denoted by an asterisk (*) and a summary of their radiological signs is to be found in Part 2 of the book. In this section conditions are listed alphabetically.

Abbreviations

ACTH	Adrenocorticotrophic hormone
AP	Anteroposterior
ASD	Atrial septal defect
AV	Atrioventricular
CMCJ	Carpometacarpal joint
CMV	Cytomegalovirus
CNS	Central nervous system
CSF	Cerebrospinal fluid
CT	Computerized tomography
CXR	Chest X-ray
DIC	Disseminated intravascular coagulopathy
DIPJ	Distal interphalangeal joint
HOA	Hypertrophic osteoarthropathy
HOCM	Hypertrophic obstructive cardiomyopathy
IAM	Internal auditory meatus
IVU	Intravenous urogram
LAT	Lateral
MCPJ	Metacarpophalangeal joint
PA	Postero-anterior
PAS	Periodic acid-Schiff (stain)
PDA	Patent ductus arteriosus
PIPJ	Proximal interphalangeal joint
PMF	Progressive massive fibrosis
PPH	Post-partum haemorrhage
SIJ	Sacroiliac joint
SLE	Systemic lupus erythematosus
SOL	Space occupying lesion
SXR	Skull X-ray
TAPVD	Total anomalous pulmonary venous drainage
TB	Tuberculosis
VSD	Ventricular septal defect

PART 1

Chapter 1
Bones

1.1 Retarded Skeletal Maturation
(Decreased Bone Age)

Generalized
1. **Severe constitutional diseases** — e.g. congenital heart disease or chronic renal failure.
2. **Cretinism*** — with granular, fragmented epiphyses.
3. **Chronic malnutrition**.
4. **Steroid therapy and Cushing's disease** — see Cushing's syndrome*.
5. **Hypopituitarism** — with growth hormone deficiency.
6. **Hypogonadism** — e.g. Turner's syndrome*.
7. **Rickets***.
8. **Congenital syndromes** — e.g. mucopolysaccharidoses and mucolipidoses.

Localized
1. **Avascular necrosis** (q.v.) — with premature fusion of the growth plate.

1.2 Accelerated Skeletal Maturation
(Increased Bone Age)

Generalized
1. **Adrenogenital syndrome** — due to adrenocortical hyperplasia or tumour.
2. **Excessive androgen or oestrogen administration or production** — e.g. adrenal or gonadal tumours.
3. **Intracranial masses, hydrocephalus and encephalitis**.
4. **McCune–Albright syndrome** — polyostotic fibrous dysplasia with precocious puberty.

Localized
1. **Inflammatory arthritides** — especially juvenile chronic arthritides.
2. **Haemophilia***.
3. **Chronic infections**.
4. **Adjacent vascular abnormality** — e.g. an arteriovenous fistula.

1.3   Dwarfism

Short Proximal Limb Bones (Rhizomelic)
1. **Achondroplasia*** — metaphyseal cupping.
2. **Thanatophoric dwarfism** — long narrow thorax, platyspondyly and curved long bones with flared and cupped metaphyses.
3. **Achondrogenesis** — severely impaired or absent mineralization of bone. Long bones not bowed. Irregular flaring of metaphyses.
4. **Metatropic dwarfism** — marked metaphyseal flaring (dumb-bell bones). Rhizomelic shortening with normal trunk at birth; later kyphoscoliosis with relatively long-limb bones.

Short Distal Limb Bones (Acromelic)
1. **Chondroectodermal dysplasia (Ellis–van Creveld syndrome)** — hypoplastic lateral tibial plateau, ulnar side polydactyly, syndactyly and carpal coalition.
2. **Asphyxiating thoracic dysplasia of Jeune** — narrow thorax with short hypoplastic ribs leading to respiratory distress. Flared ilia with inferolateral projections at the sciatic notch. Occasionally polydactyly.

Short Trunk
1. **Spondyloepiphyseal dysplasia** — oval flattened vertebrae with narrow disc spaces. Flattened epiphyses with delayed mineralization.

Short Trunk and Short Limbs
1. **Hurler's syndrome***.
2. **Hunter's syndrome** — see Hurler's syndrome*.

1.4 Lethal Neonatal Dwarfism

1. **Thanatophoric dwarfism**.
2. **Achondrogenesis**.
3. **Achondroplasia*** — especially the offspring of two achon-droplastic parents.
4. **Osteogenesis imperfecta congenita***.
5. **Hypophosphatasia***.
6. **Chondrodysplasia punctata** — rhizomelic type.
7. **Asphyxiating thoracic dysplasia of Jeune**.
8. **Campomelic dwarfism**.

1.5 Generalized Increased Bone Density — Children

Congenital
1. **Osteopetrosis** — all bones are affected and show loss of corticomedullary differentiation. Sclerosis begins as trans-verse linear densities in the metaphyses, especially notice-able in the iliac wings. Impaired modelling results in Erlenmeyer-flask-shaped long bones. Bones are brittle and heal with a normal amount of callus. Thickened base of skull with obliteration of the basal foraminae leads to deafness, optic atrophy and hydrocephalus. Obliteration of sinuses. Encroachment of marrow spaces leads to extra-medullary haemopoiesis, including hepatosplenomegaly.
2. **Engelmann's disease (progressive diaphyseal dysplasia)** — homogeneous, fusiform enlargement of the diaphyses of long bones and short tubular bones. The epiphyses and metaphyses are normal. Some narrowing of the medullary cavity with blurring of the corticomedullary junction. Occasionally, increased density of the skull base and pelvis. Muscular weakness and waddling gait.

Metabolic
1. **Renal osteodystrophy*** — rickets + osteosclerosis.

Poisoning
1. **Lead** — dense metaphyseal bands. Cortex and flat bones may also be slightly dense. Modelling deformities later, e.g. flask-shaped femora.
2. **Fluorosis** — more common in adults. Usually asymptomatic but may present in children with crippling stiffness and pain. Thickened cortex at the expense of the medulla. Periosteal reaction. Ossification of ligaments, tendons and interosseous membranes.
3. **Hypervitaminosis D** — slightly increased density of skull and vertebrae early, followed later by osteoporosis. Soft-tissue calcification. Dense metaphyseal bands and widened zone of provisional calcification.
4. **Chronic hypervitaminosis A** — not before 1 yr of age. Failure to thrive, hepatosplenomegaly, jaundice, alopecia and haemoptysis. Cortical thickening of long and tubular bones, especially in the feet. Subperiosteal new bone. Normal epiphyses and reduced metaphyseal density. The mandible is not affected (cf. Caffey's disease).

Idiopathic
1. **Caffey's disease (infantile cortical hyperostosis)** — see section 1.9.
2. **Idiopathic hypercalcaemia of infancy** — probably a manifestation of hypervitaminosis D. Elfin facies, failure to thrive and mental retardation. Generalized increased density or transverse dense metaphyseal bands. Increased density of the skull base.

1.6 Generalized Increased Bone Density — Adults

Myeloproliferative
1. **Myelosclerosis** — marrow cavity is narrowed by endosteal new bone. Patchy lucencies due to persistence of fibrous tissue. (Generalized osteopenia in the early stages due to myelofibrosis.) Hepatosplenomegaly.

Metabolic
1. **Renal osteodystrophy***.

Poisoning
1. **Fluorosis** — with periosteal reaction, prominent muscle attachments and calcification of ligaments and interosseous membranes. Changes are most marked in the innominate bones and lumbar spine.

Neoplastic (more commonly multifocal than generalized)
1. **Osteoblastic metastases** — most commonly prostate and breast. See section 1.13.
2. **Lymphoma***.
3. **Mastocytosis** — sclerosis of marrow containing skeleton with patchy areas of radiolucency. Urticaria pigmentosa. Can have symptoms and signs of carcinoid syndrome.

Idiopathic (more commonly multifocal than generalized)
1. **Paget's disease*** — coarsened trabeculae, bony expansion and thickened cortex.

Those Conditions with Onset in the Paediatric Age Group (q.v.)

1.7   Solitary Sclerotic Bone Lesion

Developmental
1. **Bone island**.
2. **Fibrous dysplasia***.

Neoplastic
1. **Metastasis** (q.v.) — most commonly prostate or breast.
2. **Lymphoma***.
3. **Osteoma/osteoid osteoma/osteoblastoma***.
4. **Healed or healing benign or malignant bone lesion** — e.g. lytic metastasis following radiotherapy or chemotherapy, bone cyst, fibrous cortical defect, eosinophilic granuloma or brown tumour.
5. **Primary bone sarcoma**.

Vascular
1. **Bone infarct** (q.v.).

Traumatic
1. **Callus** — especially a transverse density around a healing stress fracture.

Infective
1. **Sclerosing osteomyelitis of Garré**.

Idiopathic
1. **Paget's disease***.

1.8 Multiple Sclerotic Bone Lesions

Developmental
1. **Bone islands**.
2. **Fibrous dysplasia***.
3. **Osteopoikilosis** — asymptomatic. 1–10 mm, round or oval densities in the appendicular skeleton and pelvis. Ribs, skull and spine are usually exempt. Tend to be parallel to the long axis of the affected bones and are especially numerous near the ends of bones.
4. **Osteopathia striata (Voorhoeve's disease)** — asymptomatic. Linear bands of dense bone parallel with the long axis of the bone. The appendicular skeleton and pelvis are most frequently affected; skull and clavicles are spared.
5. **Tuberous sclerosis***.

Neoplastic
1. **Metastases** (q.v.) — most commonly prostate or breast.
2. **Lymphoma***.
3. **Mastocytosis**.
4. **Multiple healed or healing benign or malignant bone lesions** — e.g. lytic metastases following radiotherapy or chemotherapy, eosinophilic granuloma and brown tumours.
5. **Multiple myeloma*** — sclerosis in up to 3% of cases.
6. **Osteomata** — e.g. Gardner's syndrome.

Idiopathic
1. **Paget's disease***.

Vascular
1. **Bone infarcts** (q.v.).

Traumatic
1. **Callus** — around numerous fractures.

1.9   Bone Sclerosis with a Periosteal Reaction

Traumatic
1. **Healing fracture with callus**.

Neoplastic
1. **Metastasis**.
2. **Lymphoma***.
3. **Osteoid osteoma/osteoblastoma***.
4. **Osteogenic sarcoma***.
5. **Ewing's tumour***.
6. **Chondrosarcoma***.

Infective
1. **Osteomyelitis** — including Garré's sclerosing osteomyelitis and Brodie's abscess.
2. **Syphilis** — congenital or acquired.

Idiopathic
1. **Infantile cortical hyperostosis (Caffey's disease)** — in infants up to 6 months of age. Multiple bones involved at different times, most frequently mandible, ribs and clavicles; long bones less commonly; spine, hands and feet are spared. Increased density of bones is due to massive periosteal new bone. In the long bones the epiphyses and metaphyses are spared.
2. **Melorheostosis** — cortical and periosteal new bone giving the appearance of molten wax flowing down a burning candle. The hyperostosis tends to extend from one bone to the next. Usually affects one limb but both limbs on one side may be affected. Sometimes it is bilateral but asymmetrical. Skull, spine and ribs are seldom affected.

1.10 Solitary Sclerotic Bone Lesion with a Lucent Centre

Neoplastic
1. **Osteoid osteoma***.
2. **Osteoblastoma***.

Infective
1. **Brodie's abscess**.

1.11 Coarse Trabecular Pattern

1. **Paget's disease*** — an enlarged bone with a thickened cortex. If only part of the bone is affected the demarcation between normal and pagetoid bone is clear cut.
2. **Osteoporosis** (see   resorption of secondary trabeculae
   section 1.26)   accentuates the remaining primary
3. **Osteomalacia***   trabeculae.
4. **Haemoglobinopathies** — especially thalassaemia*.
5. **Haemangioma** — especially in a vertebral body.
6. **Gaucher's disease**.

1.12 Excessive Callus Formation

1. **Steroid therapy and Cushing's syndrome***.
2. **Neuropathic arthropathy***.
3. **Osteogenesis imperfecta***.
4. **Non-accidental injury***.
5. **Paralytic states**.
6. **Renal osteodystrophy***.
7. **Multiple myeloma***.

1.13 Skeletal Metastases — Most Common Radiological Appearances

Lung
1. **Carcinoma**	lytic
2. **Carcinoid**	sclerotic

Breast   lytic or mixed

Genito-urinary
1. **Renal cell carcinoma**	lytic, expansile
2. **Wilms' tumour**	lytic
3. **Bladder** (transitional cell)	lytic, occasionally sclerotic
4. **Prostate**	sclerotic

Reproductive Organs
1. **Cervix**	lytic or mixed
2. **Uterus**	lytic
3. **Ovary**	lytic
4. **Testis**	lytic; occasionally sclerotic

Thyroid   lytic, expansile

Gastrointestinal Tract
1. **Stomach**	sclerotic or mixed
2. **Colon**	lytic; occasionally sclerotic
3. **Rectum**	lytic

Adrenal
1. **Phaeochromocytoma**	lytic, expansile
2. **Carcinoma**	lytic
3. **Neuroblastoma**	lytic; occasionally sclerotic

Skin
1. **Squamous cell carcinoma**	lytic
2. **Melanoma**	lytic, expansile

1.14 Sites of Origin of Primary Bone Neoplasms

(A composite diagram modified from Madewell et al., 1981.)

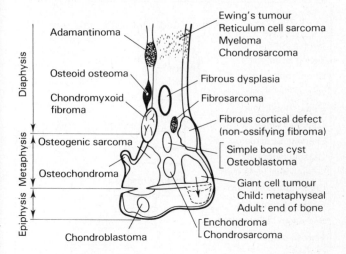

Further Reading

Madewell J.E., Ragsdale B.D. & Sweet D.E. (1981) Radiologic and pathologic analysis of solitary bone lesions. *Radiol. Clin. North Am.*, 19: 715–48.

1.15   Peak Age Incidence of Primary Bone Neoplasms

Decades	1st	2nd	3rd	4th	5th	6th	7th
Simple bone cyst							
Ewing's tumour							
Chondroblastoma							
Non-ossifying fibroma							
Osteochondroma							
Osteoblastoma							
Osteogenic sarcoma							
Osteoid osteoma							
Aneurysmal bone cyst							
Chondromyxoid fibroma							
Giant cell tumour							
Reticulum cell sarcoma							
Fibrosarcoma							
Osteoma							
Parosteal sarcoma							
Chondroma							
Haemangioma							
Chondrosarcoma							
Myeloma							
Chordoma							

1.16 Lucent Bone Lesion in the Medulla — Well-defined, Marginal Sclerosis, No Expansion

Indicates a slowly progressing lesion.

1. **Geode** — a subarticular cyst. Other signs of an arthritis. See section 1.21.
2. **Healing benign or malignant bone lesion** — e.g. metastasis, eosinophilic granuloma or brown tumour.
3. **Brodie's abscess**.
4. **Benign bone neoplasms**
   (a) Simple bone cyst* — 75% arise in the proximal humerus and femur.
   (b) Enchondroma* — more than 50% are found in the tubular bones of the hands. ± internal calcification.
   (c) Chondroblastoma* — in an epiphysis. Most common sites are proximal humerus, distal femur and proximal tibia. Internal hazy calcification.
5. **Fibrous dysplasia***.

1.17 Lucent Bone Lesion in the Medulla — Well-defined, No Marginal Sclerosis, No Expansion

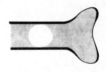

The absence of reactive bone formation implies a fast growth rate.

1. **Metastasis** — especially from breast, bronchus, kidney or thyroid.
2. **Multiple myeloma***.
3. **Eosinophilic granuloma***.
4. **Brown tumour of hyperparathyroidism***.
5. **Benign bone neoplasms**
   (a) Enchondroma*.
   (b) Chondroblastoma*.

1.18   Lucent Bone Lesion in the Medulla — Ill-defined

An aggressive pattern of destruction.

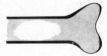

1. **Metastasis**.
2. **Multiple myeloma***.
3. **Osteomyelitis**.
4. **Lymphoma***.
5. **Long-bone sarcomas**
    (a) Osteogenic sarcoma*.
    (b) Ewing's tumour*.
    (c) Chondrosarcoma*.
    (d) Fibrosarcoma.
    (e) Reticulum cell sarcoma.

1.19 Lucent Bone Lesion in the Medulla — Well-defined, Eccentric Expansion

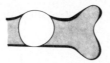

1. **Giant cell tumour*** — typically subarticular after epiphyseal fusion. (3% are metaphyseal prior to fusion). Ill-defined margins. Septa. ± soft-tissue extension and destroyed cortex. Mostly long bones.
2. **Aneurysmal bone cyst*** — in the unfused metaphysis or metaphysis and epiphysis following fusion of the growth plate. Intact but thin cortex. Well-defined endosteal margin. ± thin internal strands of bone.
3. **Enchondroma*** — diaphyseal. Over 50% occur in the tubular bones of the hands and feet. Internal ground glass appearance ± calcification within it. May be multilocular in long bones.
4. **Non-ossifying fibroma (fibrous cortical defect)*** — frequently in the distal tibia or femur and produces an eccentric expanded cortex. (In a thin bone such as the fibula central expansion is observed.) Metaphyseal. Smooth, sharp margins with a thin rim of surrounding sclerosis.
5. **Chondromyxoid fibroma*** — 75% in the lower limbs (50% in the proximal tibia). Metaphyseal and may extend into the epiphysis. Frequently has marginal sclerosis.

1.20   Lucent Bone Lesion — Grossly Expansile

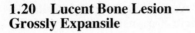

Malignant Bone Neoplasms
1. **Metastases** — renal cell carcinoma and thyroid; less commonly melanoma, bronchus, breast and phaeochromocytoma.
2. **Plasmacytoma*** — ± soft-tissue extension. ± internal septa.
3. **Chondrosarcoma/reticulum cell sarcoma/fibrosarcoma** — when slow growing may have this appearance.

Benign Bone Neoplasms
1. **Aneurysmal bone cyst*** — in the unfused metaphysis or metaphysis and epiphysis following fusion of the growth plate. ± internal septa.
2. **Giant cell tumour*** — typically subarticular after epiphyseal fusion. Ill-defined endosteal margin. ± soft-tissue extension and destroyed cortex.
3. **Endochondroma*** — ground-glass appearance ± internal calcifications.

Non-neoplastic
1. **Fibrous dysplasia*** — ground-glass appearance ± internal calcification. Modelling deformities of affected bone.
2. **Haemophilic pseudotumour** (see Haemophilia*) — especially in the iliac wing and lower limb bones. Soft-tissue swelling. ± haemophilic arthropathy.
3. **Brown tumour of hyperparathyroidism*** — the solitary skeletal sign of hyperparathyroidism in 3% of patients. Most commonly in the mandible, followed by pelvis, ribs and femora. Usually unilocular.
4. **Hydatid**.

1.21 Subarticular Lucent Bone Lesion

Arthritides
1. **Osteoarthritis** — may be multiple 'cysts' in the load-bearing areas of multiple joints. Surrounding sclerotic margin. Joint-space narrowing, subchondral sclerosis and osteophytes.
2. **Rheumatoid arthritis*** — no sclerotic margin. Begin periarticularly near the insertion of the joint capsule. Joint-space narrowing and juxta-articular osteoporosis.
3. **Calcium pyrophosphate arthropathy** (see Calcium pyrophosphate dihydrate deposition disease*) — similar to osteoarthritis but frequently larger and with more collapse and fragmentation of the articular surface.
4. **Gout*** — ± erosions with overhanging edges and adjacent soft-tissue masses.

Neoplastic
1. **Metastases/multiple myeloma*** — single or multiple. Variable appearance.
2. **Aneurysmal bone cyst*** — solitary. Expansile. Narrow zone of transition.
3. **Giant cell tumour*** — solitary. Eccentric. Ill-defined endosteal margin.
4. **Chondroblastoma*** — solitary. Predilection for the proximal ends of the humerus, femur and tibia. Contains amorphous or spotty calcification in 50%.
5. **Pigmented villonodular synovitis** — mainly the lower limb, especially the knee. Soft-tissue mass. Cyst-like defects with sharp sclerotic margins. May progress to joint destruction.

Others
1. **Post-traumatic** — particularly in the carpal bones. Well defined.
2. **Osteonecrosis** (q.v.) — with bone sclerosis, collapse and fragmentation. Preservation of joint space.
3. **Tuberculosis** — wholly epiphyseal or partly metaphyseal. Well defined or ill-defined. No surrounding sclerosis.

1.22   Lucent Bone Lesion — Containing Calcium or Bone

Neoplastic
1. **Metastases** — especially from breast.
2. **Cartilage neoplasms**
   (a) Benign — enchondroma, chondroblastoma and chondromyxoid fibroma.
   (b) Malignant — chondrosarcoma.
3. **Bone (osteoid) neoplasms**
   (a) Benign — osteoid osteoma and osteoblastoma.
   (b) Malignant — osteogenic sarcoma.
4. **Fibrous-tissue neoplasms**
   (a) Malignant — fibrosarcoma.

Others
1. **Fibrous dysplasia***.
2. **Osteoporosis circumscripta***.
3. **Osteomyelitis** — with sequestrum.
4. **Eosinophilic granuloma***.

1.23   'Moth-eaten Bone'

Multiple scattered lucencies of variable size with no major central lesion. Coalescence may occur later. Cancellous and/or cortical bone is involved.

Neoplastic
1. **Metastases** — including neuroblastoma in a child.
2. **Multiple myeloma***.
3. **Leukaemia and lymphoma***.
4. **Long-bone sarcomas**
   (a) Ewing's tumour***.
   (b) Reticulum cell sarcoma.
   (c) Osteogenic sarcoma***.
   (d) Chondrosarcoma***.
   (e) Fibrosarcoma.
5. **Histiocytosis X*** — especially in older patients.

Infective
1. **Osteomyelitis.**

1.24   Regional Osteopenia

Decreased bone density confined to a region or segment of the appendicular skeleton.

1. **Disuse** — during the immobilization of fractures, in paralysed segments and in bone and joint infections. Usually appears after 8 weeks of immobilization. The patterns of bone loss may be uniform (commonest), spotty (mostly periarticular), band-like (subchondral or metaphyseal) or endosteal cortical scalloping and linear cortical lucencies.
2. **Sudeck's atrophy (reflex sympathetic dystrophy syndrome)** — is mediated via a neurovascular mechanism and associated with post-traumatic and post-infective states, myocardial infarction, calcific tendinitis and cervical spondylosis. It most commonly affects the shoulder and hand and develops rapidly. Pain and soft-tissue swelling are clinical findings. In addition to the radiological signs of disuse there may be subperiosteal bone resorption and small periarticular erosions.
3. **Transient osteoporosis of the hip** — a severe, progressive osteoporosis of the femoral head and, to a lesser degree, of the femoral neck and acetabulum. Full recovery is seen in 6 months.
4. **Regional migratory osteoporosis** — pain, swelling and osteoporosis affect the joints of the lower limbs in particular. The migratory nature differentiates it from other causes.

1.25   Generalized Osteopenia

1. **Osteoporosis** — diminished quantity of normal bone.
2. **Osteomalacia*** — normal quantity of bone but it has an excess of uncalcified osteoid.
3. **Hyperparathyroidism*** — increased bone resorption by osteoclasts.
4. **Diffuse infiltrative bone disease** — e.g. multiple myeloma and leukaemia.

1.26   Osteoporosis

1. Decreased bone density.
2. Cortical thinning with a relative increase in density of the cortex and vertebral end-plates. Skull sutures are relatively sclerotic.
3. Relative accentuation of trabecular stress lines because of resorption of secondary trabeculae.
4. Brittle bones with an increased incidence of fractures, especially compression fractures of vertebral bodies, femoral neck and wrist fractures.

Endocrine
1. **Hypogonadism**
    (a) Ovarian — menopausal, Turner's syndrome*.
    (b) Testicular — eunuchoidism.
2. **Cushing's syndrome***.
3. **Diabetes mellitus**.
4. **Acromegaly***.
5. **Addison's disease**.
6. **Hyperthyroidism**.

Disuse

Iatrogenic
1. **Steroids***.
2. **Heparin**.

Deficiency States
1. **Vitamin C (scurvy*)**.
2. **Protein**.

Idiopathic
1. **In young people** — a rare self-limiting condition occurring in children of 8–12 years. Spontaneous improvement is seen.

Congenital
1. **Osteogenesis imperfecta***.
2. **Turner's syndrome***.
3. **Homocystinuria***.
4. **Neuromuscular diseases**.
5. **Mucopolysaccharidoses**.
6. **Trisomy 13 and 18**.
7. **Pseudo- and pseudopseudohypoparathyroidism***.
8. **Glycogen storage diseases**.
9. **Progeria**.

1.27   Osteomalacia and Rickets*

Vitamin-D Deficiency
1. **Dietary**.
2. **Malabsorption**.

Renal Disease
1. **Glomerular disease (renal osteodystrophy*)**.
2. **Renal tubular disease**
   (a) Fanconi syndromes.
   (b) X-linked hypophosphataemia.
   (c) Renal tubular acidosis.

Hepatic Disease
1. **Parenchymal failure**.
2. **Obstructive jaundice** — especially congenital biliary atresia.

Anticonvulsants
1. **Phenytoin and phenobarbitone**.

Tumour Associated
1. **Soft tissues** — haemangiopericytoma.
2. **Bone** — non-ossifying fibroma, giant cell tumour, osteo-blastoma (and fibrous dysplasia).

Not Related to Vitamin-D Metabolism
1. **Hypophosphatasia*** — low serum alkaline phosphatase.
2. **Metaphyseal chondrodysplasia (type Schmid)** — normal serum phosphate, calcium and alkaline phosphatase differentiate it from other rachitic syndromes.

If the patient is less than 6 months of age consider:
1. **Biliary atresia**.
2. **Hypophosphatasia***.
3. **Neonatal rickets** — in premature infants because of combined dietary deficiency and impaired hepatic hydroxylation of vitamin D.
4. **Vitamin D dependent rickets** — rachitic changes are associated with a severe myopathy in spite of adequate dietary intake of vitamin D. Deformed tarsal and carpal bones and platyspondyly.

1.28 Periosteal Reactions — Types

(Modified from Ragsdale et al., 1981.)

Continuous		***Interrupted***
Cortex destroyed	Intact cortex	

Shell – 'expanded cortex'

Solid smooth or undulating

Buttress

Lobulated shell

Solid spiculated

Ridged shell – 'trabeculated' 'soap bubble'

Single lamina

Codman triangle single lamina

Lamellated

Codman triangle lamellated

Parallel spiculated – 'hair-on-end'

Spiculated

Divergent spiculated – 'sunray'

The different types are, in general, non-specific, having multiple aetiologies. However, the following comments can be made:

Continuous with Destroyed Cortex
This is the result of an expanding lesion. See sections 1.19 and 1.20.

Parallel Spiculated ('Hair-on-end')
1. **Ewing's tumour***.
2. **Syphilis**.
3. **Infantile cortical hyperostosis (Caffey's disease)**.

See section 11.11 for causes in the skull vault.

Divergent Spiculated ('Sunray')
1. **Osteogenic sarcoma***.
2. **Metastases** — especially from sigmoid colon and rectum.
3. **Ewing's tumour***.
4. **Haemangioma***.
5. **Meningioma**.
6. **Tuberculosis**.
7. **Tropical ulcer**.

Codman Triangle (Single Lamina or Lamellated)
1. **Aggressive malignant tissue extending into the soft tissues**.
2. **Infection** — occasionally.

Further Reading
Ragsdale B.D., Madewell J.E. & Sweet D.E. (1981) Radiologic and pathologic analysis of solitary bone lesions. Part II: Periosteal reactions. *Radiol. Clin. North Am.*, 19: 749–83.

1.29 Periosteal Reaction — Solitary and Localized

1. **Traumatic**.
2. **Inflammatory**.
3. **Neoplastic**
   (a) Malignant
       — primary.
       — secondary.
   (b) Benign — an expanding shell or complicated by a fracture.

1.30   Periosteal Reactions — Bilaterally Symmetrical in Adults

1. **Hypertrophic osteoarthropathy (HOA)** — clinically there is clubbing of the fingers and painful swelling of knees, ankles, wrists, elbows and metacarpophalangeal joints. The periosteal reaction occurs in the metaphysis and diaphysis of the radius, ulna, tibia, fibula and, less commonly, the humerus, femur and tubular bones of the hands and feet. It can be a single lamina, lamellated or solid and undulating. Periarticular osteoporosis, soft-tissue swelling and joint effusions are other features. The condition can be caused by the conditions in section 1.31. (q.v.).

2. **Pachydermoperiostosis** — a rare, self-limiting and familial condition, usually affecting boys at puberty and with a predilection for blacks. Clinically there is an insidious onset of thickening of the skin of the extremities (including the face), hyperhidrosis and clubbing. Compared with HOA it is relatively pain free. The bones most commonly affected are the tibia, fibula, radius and ulna (less commonly the carpus, tarsus and tubular bones of the hands and feet). The periosteal reaction is similar to HOA but is more solid and spiculated and also involves the epiphysis to produce outgrowths around joints. The concavity of the diaphysis may be filled in. ± ligamentous calcification.

3. **Vascular insufficiency (venous, lymphatic or arterial)** — the legs are almost exclusively affected with involvement of tibia, fibula, metatarsals and phalanges. There is a solid undulating periosteal reaction, which is, initially, separated from the cortex but later merges with it. No definite relationship to soft-tissue ulceration. Phleboliths may be associated with venous stasis. Soft-tissue swelling is a feature whatever the aetiology. Arterial insufficiency due to polyarteritis nodosa or other arteritides may also be associated with a mild periostitis and is also usually confined to the lower limbs.

4. **Thyroid acropachy** — in 0.5–10% of patients following thyroidectomy for thyrotoxicosis and who may now be euthyroid, hypothyroid or hyperthyroid. Clinically there is soft-tissue swelling, clubbing, exophthalmos and pretibial myxoedema. A solid, spiculated, almost lace-like periosteal reaction affects the diaphysis of the metacarpals and phalanges of the hands, especially the radial side of the thumbs and index fingers. Less commonly the feet, lower legs and forearms are involved.
5. **Fluorosis** — solid, undulating periosteal reaction with osteosclerosis. The long bones and tubular bones are most frequently affected. Ligamentous calcification.

1.31 Hypertrophic Osteoarthropathy

Pulmonary
1. **Carcinoma of bronchus**.
2. **Lymphoma***.
3. **Abscess**.
4. **Bronchiectasis**.
5. **Metastases**.

Pleural
1. **Pleural fibroma** — has the highest incidence of accompanying HOA, although it is itself a rare cause.
2. **Mesothelioma**.

Cardiovascular
1. **Cyanotic congenital heart disease** — produces clubbing but only rarely a periosteal reaction.

Gastrointestinal
1. **Ulcerative colitis***.
2. **Crohn's disease***.
3. **Dysentery** — amoebic or bacillary.
4. **Lymphoma***.
5. **Whipple's disease**.
6. **Coeliac disease**.
7. **Cirrhosis** — especially primary biliary cirrhosis.
8. **Nasopharyngeal carcinomas (Schmincke's tumour)**.

1.32   Periosteal Reactions — Bilaterally Symmetrical in Children

1. **Normal premature infants** — up to 4 months of age and due to minimal trauma.
2. **Juvenile chronic arthritis*** — in approx 25% of cases. Most common in the periarticular regions of the pha-langes, metacarpals and metatarsals. When it extends into the diaphysis it will eventually result in enlarged, rect-angular tubular bones.
3. **Acute leukaemia** — associated with prominent metaphyseal bone resorption ± a dense zone of provisional calcification. Osteopenia. Periosteal reaction is due to cortical involve-ment by tumour cells. Metastatic neuroblastoma can look identical.
4. **Scurvy*** — subperiosteal haemorrhage is most frequent in the femur, tibia and humerus. Periosteal reaction is particularly evident during the healing phase. Age 6 months or older.
5. **Congenital syphilis** — an exuberant periosteal reaction can be due to infiltration by syphilitic granulation tissue or the healing (with callus formation) of osteochondritis. The former is essentially diaphyseal and the latter around the metaphyseal/epiphyseal junction.
6. **Caffey's disease** — first evident before 5 months of age. Mandible, clavicles and ribs show cortical hyperostosis and a diffuse periosteal reaction. The scapulae and tubular bones are less often affected and tend to be involved asymmetrically.
7. **Rickets*** — the presence of uncalcified subperiosteal osteoid *mimics* a periosteal reaction because the perio-steum and ossified cortex are separated.

1.33 Periosteal Reactions — Bilaterally Asymmetrical

1. **Metastases**.
2. **Osteomyelitis**.
3. **Arthritides** — especially Reiter's syndrome* and psoriatic arthropathy*.
4. **Osteoporosis** (q.v.) ⎫ because of the increased
5. **Osteomalacia** (q.v.) ⎭ liability to fractures.
6. **Non-accidental injury***.
7. **Bleeding diatheses**.
8. **Hand–foot syndrome (sickle-cell dactylitis)** — see Sickle-cell anaemia*.

1.34 Pseudarthrosis

1. **Non-union of a fracture**.
2. **Congenital** — in the middle to lower third of the tibia ± fibula. 50% present in the first year. Later there is cupping of the proximal bone end and pointing of the distal bone end.
3. **Neurofibromatosis***.
4. **Osteogenesis imperfecta***.
5. **Cleidocranial dysplasia*** — congenitally in the femur.
6. **Fibrous dysplasia***.
7. **Ankylosing spondylitis*** — in the fused bamboo spine.

Further Reading
Boyd H.B. & Sage F.P. (1958) Congenital pseudarthrosis of the tibia. *J. Bone Joint Surg.*, 40A: 1245–70.
Park W.M., Spencer D.G., McCall I.W., Ward D.J., Watson Buchanan W. & Stephens W.H. (1981) The detection of spinal pseudarthrosis in ankylosing spondylitis. *Br. J. Radiol.*, 54: 467–72.

1.35   Irregular or Stippled Epiphyses

1. **Avascular necrosis** (q.v.) — single, e.g. Perthes' disease (although 10% are bilateral), or multiple, e.g. sickle-cell anaemia.
2. **Cretinism*** — not present at birth. Delayed appearance and growth of ossification centres. Appearance varies from slightly granular to fragmentation. The femoral capital epiphysis may be divided into inner and outer halves.
3. **Morquio's syndrome*** — irregular ossification of the femoral capital epiphyses results in flattening.
4. **Multiple epiphyseal dysplasia** — onset 5–14 years. May be familial. Delayed appearance and growth of epiphyses but the time of fusion is normal. ± metaphyseal irregularity. Carpal and tarsal bones, hips, knees and ankles are most commonly affected. Tibio-talar slant. Short, stubby digits and metacarpals. Spine usually, but not always, normal. Early and severe osteoarthritis.
5. **Chondrodysplasia punctata** — stippling occurs prior to the normal time of appearance of the epiphysis. Hips, knees, shoulders and wrists are most commonly affected. The abnormality may disappear by 3 years of age. Stippled laryngeal calcification. Wormian bones. There are two types:
   (a) Rhizomelic — usually die in the first year. Symmetrical long-bone shortening.
   (b) Conradi–Hünermann — survive. Asymmetrical limb shortening.
6. **Trisomy 18 and 21**.
7. **Prenatal infections**.

1.36 Avascular Necrosis

Toxic
1. **Steroids*** — probably does not occur with less than 2 years of treatment.
2. **Anti-inflammatory drugs** — indomethacin and phenyl-butazone.
3. **Alcohol** — possibly because of fat emboli in chronic alcoholic pancreatitis.
4. **Immunosuppressives**.

Traumatic
1. **Idiopathic** — e.g. Perthes' disease and other osteochondritides.
2. **Fractures** — especially femoral neck, talus and scaphoid.
3. **Radiotherapy**.
4. **Heat** — burns.
5. **Fat embolism**.

Inflammatory
1. **Rheumatoid arthritis***.   } in the absence of drugs
2. **Systemic lupus erythematosus***. } probably due to a vasculitis.
3. **Scleroderma***.
4. **Infection** — e.g. following a pyogenic arthritis.
5. **Pancreatitis**.

Metabolic and Endocrine
1. **Pregnancy**.
2. **Diabetes**.
3. **Cushing's syndrome***.
4. **Hyperlipidaemias**.
5. **Gout***.

Haemopoietic Disorders
1. **Haemoglobinopathies** — especially sickle-cell anaemia*.
2. **Polycythaemia rubra vera**.
3. **Gaucher's disease**.
4. **Haemophilia***.

Thrombotic and Embolic
1. **Dysbaric osteonecrosis**.
2. **Arteritis**.

1.37   Supernumerary Epiphyseal Ossification Centres

1. **Idiopathic.**
2. **Cleidocranial dysplasia*.**
3. **Down's syndrome*.**
4. **Cretinism*.**

1.38   The Abnormal Metaphysis (excluding metaphyseal dysplasias)

see table pages 36 and 37.

1.39   Erosion or Absence of the Outer End of the Clavicle

1. **Rheumatoid arthritis*.**
2. **Hyperparathyroidism*.**
3. **Multiple myeloma*.**
4. **Metastasis.**
5. **Post-traumatic osteolysis.**
6. **Cleidocranial dysplasia*.**

1.40   Focal Rib Lesion (Solitary or Multiple)

Neoplastic
Secondary more common than primary.
Primary malignant more common than benign.
1. **Metastases**
    (a) **Adult male** — bronchus, kidney or prostate most commonly.
    (b) **Adult female** — breast.
    (c) **Child** — neuroblastoma.
2. **Primary malignant**
    (a) **Multiple myeloma/plasmacytoma*.**
    (b) **Chondrosarcoma*.**
    (c) **Ewing's tumour*** — in a child.
3. **Benign**
    (a) **Osteochondroma*.**
    (b) **Enchondroma*.**
    (c) **Histiocytosis X*.**

Non-neoplastic
1. **Healed rib fracture.**
2. **Fibrous dysplasia*.**
3. **Paget's disease*.**
4. **Brown tumour of hyperparathyroidism*.**
5. **Osteomyelitis** — bacterial, tuberculous or fungal.

Further Reading
Omell G.H., Anderson L.S. & Bramson R.T. (1973) Chest wall tumours. *Radiol. Clin. North Am.*, 11: 197–214.

| | Epiphysis | Growth plate | METAPHYSIS | | |
			Zone of provisional calcification	Widening	Fraying
Congenital rubella / Congenital CMV	Ill defined	N	Absent	−	Celery stick
Congenital syphilis	N	Wide	Wide	+	+
Cretinism	Irregular	N	Dense	−	−
Osteopetrosis	Dense	N	Dense	+	−
Phenylketonuria	Retarded	Spicules of calcification from metaphysis	N	−	spiculated
Rickets	Ill defined	Wide	Early — ill defined Healing — wide and dense	+	+
Scurvy	Ringed	Narrow	Wide and dense	After fracture	−
Heavy metal poisoning	N	N	+	+	−
Leukaemia / Secondary neuroblastoma	Normal or ill defined	N	N or dense if treated with folic acid	−	−
Chronic hypervitaminosis A	May be enlarged	N	Wide	+	+
Hypervitaminosis D	N	N	Wide	−	−
Non-accidental injury	N	N	N	After fracture	−
Growth arrest lines	N	N	N	−	−

N = Normal;   + = Present;   − = Absent.

| | METAPHYSIS | | | | |
Cupping	Lucent band	Other dense bands	Fracture	Periosteal reaction	Age at onset
−	+	−	−	−	Birth
+	+	−	+	+	Birth
−	−	+	−	−	Birth
+	−	+	−	−	Birth
+	−	−	−	−	1 month
+	−	Treatment	−	+	6 months
After fracture	+	−	+	+	6 months
−	−	If intermittent exposure	−	−	After 1 year
−	+	−	−	+	2–5 years
+	−	−	−	+	1–3 years
−	+	+	−	−	Variable
Late	−	−	+	+	Variable
−	−	+	−	−	Variable

1.41   Rib Notching — Inferior Surface

Arterial
1. **Coarctation of the aorta** — rib signs are unusual before 10 years of age. Affects 4–8th ribs bilaterally; not the upper two if conventional. Unilateral and right-sided if the coarctation is proximal to the left subclavian artery. Unilateral and left-sided if associated with an anomalous right subclavian artery distal to the coarctation. Other signs include a prominent ascending aorta and a small descending aorta with an intervening notch, left ventricular enlargement and possibly signs of heart failure.
2. **Aortic thrombosis** — usually the lower ribs bilaterally.
3. **Subclavian obstruction** — most commonly post Blalock operation (either subclavian-to-pulmonary artery anastomosis) for Fallot's tetralogy. Unilateral rib notching of the upper three or four ribs on the operation side.
4. **Pulmonary oligaemia** — any cause of decreased pulmonary blood supply.

Venous
1. **Superior vena caval obstruction**.

Arteriovenous
1. **Pulmonary arteriovenous malformation**.
2. **Chest wall arteriovenous malformation**.

Neurogenic
1. **Neurofibromatosis*** — 'ribbon ribs' may also be a feature.

1.42 Rib Notching — Superior Surface

Connective Tissue Diseases
1. **Rheumatoid arthritis***.
2. **Systemic lupus erythematosus***.
3. **Scleroderma***.
4. **Sjögren's syndrome**.

Metabolic
1. **Hyperparathyroidism***.

Miscellaneous
1. **Neurofibromatosis***.
2. **Restrictive lung disease**.
3. **Poliomyelitis**.
4. **Marfan's syndrome***.
5. **Osteogenesis imperfecta***.
6. **Progeria**.

1.43 Arachnodactyly

Elongated and slender tubular bones of the hands and feet. The metacarpal index is an aid to diagnosis and is estimated by measuring the lengths of the 2nd, 3rd, 4th and 5th metacarpals and dividing by their breadths taken at the exact mid-points. These four figures are then added together and divided by 4.
Normal range   5.4–7.9
Arachnodactyly range   8.4–10.4

1. **Marfan's syndrome*** — although arachnodactyly is not necessary for the diagnosis.
2. **Homocystinuria*** — morphologically resembles Marfan's syndrome but 60% are mentally defective, they have a predisposition to arterial and venous thromboses and the lens of the eye dislocates downward rather than upward.

1.44   Distal Phalangeal Resorption (Acro-osteolysis)

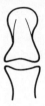 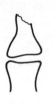

Normal   Resorption of   Resorption of   Periarticular
              the tuft   the mid portion

Resorption of the Tuft
1. **Scleroderma***.
2. **Raynaud's disease**.
3. **Psoriatic arthropathy***.
4. **Neuropathic diseases** — diabetes mellitus, leprosy, myelomeningocoele, syringomyelia and congenital indifference to pain.
5. **Thermal injuries** — burns, frostbite and electrical.
6. **Trauma**.
7. **Hyperparathyroidism***.
8. **Epidermolysis bullosa**.

Resorption of the Mid Portion
1. **Polyvinyl chloride tank cleaners**.
2. **Acro-osteolysis of Hajdu and Cheney**.
3. **Hyperparathyroidism***.

Periarticular — i.e. erosion of the distal interphalangeal joints
1. **Psoriatic arthropathy***.
2. **Erosive osteoarthritis**.
3. **Hyperparathyroidism***.
4. **Thermal injuries**.
5. **Scleroderma***.
6. **Multicentric reticulohistiocytosis**.

1.45 Short Metacarpal(s) or Metatarsal(s)

1. **Idiopathic**.
2. **Post-traumatic** — iatrogenic, fracture, growth plate injury, thermal or electrical.
3. **Post-infarction** — e.g. sickle-cell anaemia*.
4. **Turner's syndrome*** — 4th ± 3rd & 5th metacarpals.
5. **Pseudo- and pseudopseudohypoparathyroidism*** — 4th & 5th metacarpals.

1.46 Carpal Fusion

Isolated
Tends to involve bones in the same carpal row (proximal or distal). More common in Negroes than Caucasians.

1. **Triquetral–lunate** — the most common site. Affects 1% of the population.
2. **Capitate–hamate**.
3. **Trapezium–trapezoid**.

Syndrome-related
Tends to exhibit massive carpal fusion affecting bones in different rows (proximal and distal).

1. **Acrocephalosyndactyly (Apert's syndrome)**.
2. **Arthrogryposis multiplex congenita**.
3. **Ellis–van Creveld syndrome**.
4. **Holt–Oram syndrome**.
5. **Turner's syndrome***.
6. **Symphalangism**.

Acquired
1. **Inflammatory arthritides** — especially juvenile chronic arthritis* and rheumatoid arthritis*.
2. **Pyogenic arthritis**.
3. **Post-traumatic**.
4. **Post-surgical**.

Further Reading
Cope J.R. (1974) Carpal coalition. *Clin. Radiol.*, 25: 261–6.

42   Aids to Radiological Differential Diagnosis

Bibliography

General
Felson B. (ed.) (1970) The foot. *Semin. Roentgenol.*, 5(4).
Greenfield G.B. (1980) *Radiology of Bone Disease*, 3rd edn. Philadelphia: Lippincott.
Murray R.O. & Jacobson H.G. (1977) *The Radiology of Skeletal Disorders*, 2nd edn. Edinburgh: Churchill Livingstone.
Poznanski A.K. (1974) *The Hand in Radiological Diagnosis*. Philadelphia: Saunders.
Resnick D. & Niwayama G. (1981) *Diagnosis of Bone and Joint Disorders*. Philadelphia: Saunders.
Sutton D. (1980) *Textbook of Radiology and Imaging*, 3rd edn, chaps 1–10. Edinburgh: Churchill Livingstone.

Benign Neoplasms
Byers P.D. (1968) Solitary benign osteoblastic lesions of bone. *Cancer*, 22: 43–57.
Clough J.R. & Price C.H.G. (1968) Aneurysmal bone cysts. *J. Bone Joint Surg.*, 50B: 116–27.
Lodwick G.S. (1958) Juvenile unicameral bone cyst. *Am. J. Roentgenol.*, 83: 495–504.
McLeod R.A. & Beabout J.W. (1973) The roentgenographic features of chondroblastoma. *Am. J. Roentgenol.*, 118: 464–71.
Maudsley R.H. (1956) Non-osteogenic fibroma of bone (fibrous metaphyseal defect). *J. Bone Joint Surg.*, 38B: 714–33.
Murphy N.B. & Price C.H.G. (1971) The radiological aspects of chondromyxoid fibroma of bone. *Clin. Radiol.*, 22: 261–9.
Omojola M.F. Cockshott W.P. & Beatty E.G. (1981) Osteoid osteoma: an evaluation of diagnostic modalities. *Clin. Radiol.*, 32: 199–204.

Malignant Neoplasms
Barnes R. & Catto M. (1966) Chondrosarcoma of bone. *J. Bone Joint Surg.*, 48B: 729–64.
Dahlin D.C. (1967) Osteogenic sarcoma. A study of 600 cases. *J. Bone Joint Surg.*, 49A: 101–10.
Dahlin D.C., Coventry M.B. & Scanlon P.W. (1961) Ewing's sarcoma: a critical analysis of 165 cases. *J. Bone Joint Surg.*, 43A: 185–92.
Jacobs P. (1972) The diagnosis of osteoclastoma (giant cell tumour): a radiological and pathological correlation. *Br. J. Radiol.*, 45: 121–36.
Pagani J.J. & Libshitz H.I. (1982) Imaging bone metastases. *Radiol. Clin. North Am.*, 20(3): 545–60.

Infections

Chapman M., Murray R.O. & Stoker D.J. (1979) Tuberculosis of the bones and joints. *Semin. Roentgenol.*, 14: 266–82.

Cremin B.J. & Fisher R.M. (1970) The lesions of congenital syphilis. *Br. J. Radiol.*, 43: 333–41.

Enna C.D., Jacobson R.A. & Rausch R.O. (1971) Bone changes in leprosy. *Radiology*, 100: 295–306.

Goldblatt M. & Cremin B.J. (1978) Osteoarticular tuberculosis: its presentation in coloured races. *Clin. Radiol.*, 29: 669–77.

Latham W.J. (1953) Hydatid disease. *J. Faculty Radiol.*, 5: 65–81 & 83–95.

Dysplasias, etc.

Dorst J.P., Scott C.I. & Hall J.G. (1972) The radiological assessment of short-stature dwarfism. *Radiol. Clin. North Am.*, 10(3): 393–414.

Felson B. (ed.) (1973) Dwarfs and other little people. *Semin. Roentgenol.*, 8(2).

Spranger J.W., Langer L.O. & Wiedmann H.R. (1974) *Bone Dysplasias: An Atlas of Constitutional Disorders of Skeletal Development*. Philadelphia: Saunders.

Metabolic Bone Disease

Doyle F.H. (1975) Current concepts in metabolic bone disease. In: Lodge T. & Steiner R. (eds) *Recent Advances in Radiology*, No. 5. Edinburgh: Churchill Livingstone.

Grainger R.G. (1964) The radiology of metabolic bone disease. In: Lodge T. (ed.) *Recent Advances in Radiology*, No. 4. Edinburgh: Churchill Livingstone.

Ischaemia

Davidson J.K. (1979) Dysbaric osteonecrosis and pulmonary changes in divers. In: Lodge T. & Steiner R.E. (eds) *Recent Advances in Radiology and Medical Imaging — 6*, pp 145–62. Edinburgh: Churchill Livingstone.

Edeiken J., Hodes P.J., Libshitz H.I. & Weller M.H. (1967) Bone ischaemia. *Radiol. Clin. North Am.*, 5(3): 515–29.

Chapter 2
The Spine

2.1 Scoliosis

Idiopathic
1. **Infantile** — diagnosed before the age of 4 years. 90% are thoracic and concave to the right. More common in boys. 90% resolve spontaneously.
2. **Juvenile** — diagnosed between 4 and 10 years. More common in girls. Almost always progressive.
3. **Adolescent** — diagnosed between 10 years and maturity. More common in females. Majority are concave to the left in the thoracic region.

Congenital
Most common in the thoracic spine. The defects in development may be classifed as follows:

1. **Failure of formation**
   (a) Unilateral hypoplasia (wedge vertebra).
   (b) Unilateral aplasia (hemivertebra).
2. **Unilateral failure of segmentation**
   (a) Posterior elements only.
   (b) Vertebral body only.
   (c) Vertebral body and posterior elements.
3. **Partial duplication (supernumerary hemivertebra).**
4. **Combination of the above lesions.**

Associated abnormalities may occur — urinary tract (18%), congenital heart disease (7%), undescended scapulae (6%) and diastematomyelia (5%).

Neuromuscular Diseases
1. **Myelomeningocoele**.
2. **Spinal muscular atrophy**.
3. **Friedreich's ataxia**.
4. **Poliomyelitis**.
5. **Cerebral palsy**.
6. **Muscular dystrophy**.

Mesodermal and Neuroectodermal Diseases
1. **Neurofibromatosis*** — in up to 40% of patients. Classically a sharply angled short segment scoliosis with a severe kyphosis. The apical vertebrae are irregular and wedged with adjacent dysplastic ribs. 25% have a congenital vertebral anomaly.
2. **Marfan's syndrome*** — scoliosis in 40–60%. Double structural curves are typical.
3. **Homocystinuria*** — similar to Marfan's syndrome.

Post Radiotherapy
Wedged and hypoplastic vertebrae ± unilateral pelvic or rib hypoplasia.

Leg Length Discrepancy
A flexible lumbar curve, convex to the side of the shorter leg. Disparity of iliac crest level.

Painful Scoliosis
1. **Osteoid osteoma*** — 10% occur in the spine. A lamina or pedicle at the apex of the curve will be sclerotic or overgrown.
2. **Osteoblastoma***.
3. **Intraspinal tumour** (q.v.).
4. **Infection**.

2.2   Solitary Collapsed Vertebra

1. **Neoplastic disease**
    (a) Metastasis — breast, bronchus, prostate, kidney and thyroid account for the majority of patients with a solitary spinal metastasis. The disc spaces are preserved until late. The bone may be lytic, sclerotic or mixed. ± destruction of a pedicle.
    (b) Multiple myeloma/plasmacytoma* — a common site, especially for plasmacytoma. May mimic an osteolytic metastasis or be expansile and resemble an aneurysmal bone cyst.
    (c) Lymphoma*.
2. **Osteoporosis** (q.v.) — generalized osteopenia. Coarsened trabecular pattern in adjacent vertebrae due to resorption of secondary trabeculae.
3. **Trauma**.
4. **Infection** — with destruction of vertebral end-plates and adjacent disc spaces.
5. **Histiocytosis X*** — eosinophil granuloma is the most frequent cause of a solitary vertebra plana in childhood. The posterior elements are usually spared.
6. **Benign tumours** — haemangioma, giant cell tumour and aneurysmal bone cyst.

2.3 Multiple Collapsed Vertebrae

1. **Osteoporosis** (q.v.) — reduced bone density. Vertebral bodies may be wedged or biconcave (fish-shaped).
2. **Neoplastic disease** — wedge fractures are particularly related to osteolytic metastases and osteolytic marrow tumours, e.g. multiple myeloma, and lymphoma. Altered or obliterated normal trabeculae. Disc spaces are usually preserved until late. Paravertebral soft-tissue mass is more common in myeloma than metastases.
3. **Trauma** — discontinuity of trabeculae, sclerosis of the fracture line due to compressed and overlapping trabeculae. Disc space usually preserved. The lower cervical, lower dorsal and upper lumbar spine are most commonly affected. Usually no soft-tissue mass.
4. **Scheuermann's disease** — irregular end plates and numerous Schmorl's nodes in the thoracic spine of children and young adults. Disc space narrowing. Often progresses to a severe kyphosis. Secondary degenerative changes later.
5. **Infection** — destruction of end plates adjacent to a destroyed disc. Although it is usually not possible to differentiate radiologically between pyogenic and tuberculous spondylitis in white patients, the following signs are said to be helpful.

Pyogenic	Tuberculous
Rapidly progressive	Slower progression
Marked osteoblastic response	Less sclerosis
Less collapse	Marked collapse
Small or no paravertebral abscess	Large paravertebral abscess
Early bridging of affected vertebrae	

6. **Histiocytosis X*** — the spine is more frequently involved in eosinophilic granuloma and Hand–Schüller–Christian disease than in Letterer–Siwe disease. Most common in young people. The thoracic and lumbo-sacral spine are the usual sites of disease. Disc spaces are preserved.
7. **Sickle-cell anaemia*** — characteristice step-like depression in the central part of the end-plate.

Further Reading
Allen E.H., Cosgrove D. & Millard F.J.C. (1978) The radiological changes in infections of the spine and their diagnostic value. *Clin. Radiol.*, 29: 31–40.
Goldman A.B. & Freiberger R.H. (1978) Localised infections and neuropathic disease. *Semin. Roentgenol.*, 14: 19–32.

2.4   Congenital Platyspondyly

1. **Achondroplasia*** — other spinal changes include antero-inferior beaks in the thoracolumbar region, posterior scalloping and short pedicles with a narrow lumbar canal.
2. **Thanatophoric dwarfism** — long narrow thorax and curved long bones with concave irregular metaphyses. Lethal.
3. **Osteogenesis imperfecta*** — softened osteopenic bodies show symmetrical flattening or biconcavities due to ballooning of the intervertebral discs. Fractures.
4. **Cretinism*** — flattened, ovoid vertebral bodies are noted at or soon after birth. The disc spaces are wide, the neurocentral synchondroses are open and there is failure of fusion of the neural arches. Wide neural canal. In the neck prevertebral soft-tissue swelling may be present. There may be an antero-inferior beak in the thoracolumbar region.
5. **Morquio's syndrome*** — universal, flattened, elongated vertebral bodies with a central anterior beak. The superior and inferior end-plates may be roughened.
6. **Spondyloepiphyseal dysplasia**
   (a) Congenita — irregularities of the end-plates. Flattening is most marked in the thoracolumbar region and associated with a kyphoscoliosis.
   (b) Tarda — males only and evident just before puberty. Platyspondyly is greatest in the thoracic region and the vertebral bodies show characteristic new bone in the posterior two-thirds of the articular surface with depression of the anterior one-third. Premature osteoarthritis of the hips.
7. **Metatropic dwarfism** — short tongue shaped vertebral bodies with a gap in the neural arch. Later in childhood the vertebrae are less flat but there is severe kyphoscoliosis.

2.5   Erosion, Destruction or Absence of a Pedicle

1. **Metastasis**

2. **Multiple myeloma***

   metastatic carcinoma involves the pedicle relatively early and contrasts with the late preservation of the pedicle in multiple myeloma.

3. **Intraspinal mass** (q.v.) — with widening of the interpedicular distance.
4. **Tuberculosis** — uncommonly. With a large paravertebral abscess.
5. **Benign bone tumour** — aneurysmal bone cyst or giant cell tumour.
6. **Congenital absence** — ± sclerosis of the contralateral pedicle.

Further Reading

Bell D. & Cockshott W.P. (1971) Tuberculosis of the vertebral pedicle. *Radiology*, 99: 43–8.

2.6   Solitary Dense Pedicle

1. **Osteoblastic metastasis** — no change in size.
2. **Osteoid osteoma*** — some enlargement of the pedicle ± radiolucent nidus.
3. **Osteoblastoma*** — larger than osteoid osteoma and more frequently a lucency with a sclerotic margin rather than a purely sclerotic pedicle.
4. **Secondary to spondylolysis** — ipsilateral or contralateral.
5. **Secondary to congenitally absent or hypoplastic contralateral posterior elements.**

Further Reading

Wilkinson R.H. & Hall J.E. (1974) The sclerotic pedicle: tumour or pseudotumour? *Radiology*, 111: 683–8.

2.7   Enlarged Vertebral Body

Generalized
1. **Gigantism.**
2. **Acromegaly***.

Local (Single or Multiple)
1. **Paget's disease***.
2. **Benign bone tumour**
   (a) Aneurysmal bone cyst*— typically purely lytic and expansile. Involves the anterior and posterior elements more commonly than the anterior or posterior elements alone. Rapid growth.
   (b) Haemangioma* — with a prominent vertical trabecular pattern.
   (c) Giant cell tumour* — involvement of the body alone is most common. Expansion is minimal.
3. **Hydatid** — over 40% of cases of hydatid disease in bone occur in vertebrae.

Further Reading
Beabout J.W., McLeod R.A. & Dahlin D.C. (1979) Benign tumours. *Semin. Roentgenol.*, 14: 33–43.
Dahlin D.C. (1977) Giant cell tumour of vertebrae above the sacrum. A review of 31 cases. *Cancer*, 39: 1350–6.
Mohan V., Gupta S.K., Tuli S.M. & Sanyal B. (1980) Symptomatic vertebral haemangiomas. *Clin. Radiol.*, 31: 575–9.

2.8   Squaring of One or More Vertebral Bodies

1. **Ankylosing spondylitis***.
2. **Paget's disease***.
3. **Psoriatic arthropathy***.
4. **Reiter's syndrome***.
5. **Rheumatoid arthritis***.

2.9 Block Vertebrae

1. **Isolated congenital** — a failure of segmentation. Most common in the lumbar spine but also occurs in the cervical and thoracic regions. The ring epiphyses of adjacent vertebrae do not develop and thus the AP diameter of the vertebrae at the site of the segmentation defect is decreased. The articular facets, neural arches or spinous processes may also be involved. A faint lucency representing a vestigial disc may be observed.

2. **Klippel–Feil syndrome** — segmentation defects in the cervical spine, short neck, low hairline and limited cervical movement, especially rotation. The radiological appearance of the cervical spine resembles (1) above. C2–C3 and C5–C6 are most commonly affected. Other anomalies are frequently associated, the most important being
   (a) Scoliosis > 20° in more than 50% of patients.
   (b) Sprengel's shoulder in 30%, ± an omovertebral body.
   (c) Cervical ribs.
   (d) Genito-urinary abnormalities in 66%; renal agenesis in 33%.
   (e) Deafness in 33%.

3. **Rheumatoid arthritis*** — especially juvenile onset rheumatoid arthritis and juvenile chronic arthritis with polyarticular onset. There may be angulation at the fusion site and this is not a feature of the congenital variety. The spinous processes do not fuse.

4. **Ankylosing spondylitis*** — squaring of anterior vertebral margins and calcification in the intervertebral discs and anterior and posterior longitudinal ligaments.

5. **Tuberculosis** — vertebral body collapse and destruction of the disc space, ± paraspinal calcification. There may be angulation of the spine.

6. **Operative fusion**.

7. **Post-traumatic**.

2.10   Ivory Vertebral Body

Single or multiple very dense vertebrae. The list excludes those causes where increased density is due to compaction of bone following collapse. If there is generalized involvement of the spine see section 1.6.

1. **Metastases** — sclerotic metastases or an initially lytic metastasis which, after treatment, has become sclerotic. Usually no alteration in vertebral body size. Disc spaces preserved until late.
2. **Paget's disease*** — usually a single vertebral body is affected. Expanded body with a thickened cortex and coarsened trabeculation. Disc space involvement is uncommon.
3. **Lymphoma*** — more frequent in Hodgkin's disease than the other reticuloses. Normal size vertebral body. Disc spaces intact.
4. **Low-grade infection** — with end-plate destruction, disc space narrowing and a paraspinal soft-tissue mass.

2.11 Atlanto-axial Subluxation

When the distance between the posterior aspect of the anterior arch of the atlas and the anterior aspect of the odontoid process exceeds 3 mm in adults and older children or 5 mm in younger children, or an interosseous distance that changes considerably between flexion and extension.

Arthritides
1. **Rheumatoid arthritis*** — in 20–25% of patients with severe disease. Associated erosion of the odontoid may be severe enough to reduce it to a small spicule of bone.
2. **Psoriatic arthropathy*** — in 45% of patients with spondylitis.
3. **Juvenile chronic arthritis*** — most commonly in seropositive juvenile onset adult rheumatoid arthritis.
4. **Systemic lupus erythematosus***.
5. **Ankylosing spondylitis*** — in 2% of cases. Usually a late feature.

Trauma

Infection
1. **Retropharyngeal abscess in a child**.

Congenital
1. **Down's syndrome*** — in 20% of cases.
2. **Morquio's syndrome***.
3. **Congenital absence/hypoplasia of the dens** — 66% have a history of previous trauma.
4. **Atlanto-occipital fusion**.

2.12   Intervertebral Disc Calcification

1. **Degenerative spondylosis** — in the nucleus pulposus. Usually confined to the dorsal region. With other signs of degenerative spondylosis — disc-space narrowing, osteophytosis and vacuum sign in the disc. A frequent finding in the elderly.

2. **Alkaptonuria*** — symptoms of arthropathy first appear in the 4th decade. Widespread disc calcification, osteoporosis, disc-space narrowing and osteophytosis. The disc calcification is predominantly in the inner fibres of the annulus fibrosus but may be diffusely throughout the disc. Severe changes progress to ankylosis and may mimic ankylosing spondylitis.

3. **Calcium pyrophosphate dihydrate deposition disease*** — predominantly in the outer fibres of the annulus fibrosus.

4. **Ankylosing spondylitis*** — in the nucleus pulposus. Ankylosis, square vertebral bodies and syndesmophytes.

5. **Juvenile chronic arthritis*** — may mimic ankylosing spondylitis.

6. **Haemochromatosis*** — in the outer fibres of the annulus fibrosus.

7. **Diffuse idiopathic skeletal hyperostosis (DISH)** — may mimic ankylosing spondylitis.

8. **Gout***

9. **Idiopathic** — a transient phenomenon in children. The cervical spine is most often affected. Clinically associated with neck pain and fever but may be asymptomatic. Persistent in adults.

10. **Following spinal fusion**.

Further Reading

Weinberger A. & Myers A.R. (1978) Intervertebral disc calcification in adults: a review. *Semin. Arthritis Rheum.*, 18: 69–75.

2.13 Bony Outgrowths of the Spine

Syndesmophytes
Ossification of the annulus fibrosus. Thin, vertical and symmetrical. When extreme results in the 'bamboo spine'.

1. **Ankylosing spondylitis***.
2. **Alkaptonuria**.

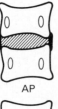

AP

Paravertebral Ossification
Ossification of paravertebral connective tissue which is separated from the edge of the vertebral body and disc. Large, coarse and asymmetrical.

1. **Reiter's syndrome***.
2. **Psoriatic arthropathy***.

AP

Claw Osteophytes
Arising from the vertebral margin with no gap and having an obvious claw appearance

1. **Stress response** — but in the absence of disc space narrowing does not indicate disc degeneration.

Lateral

Traction Spurs
Osteophytes with a gap between the end-plate and the base of the osteophyte and with the tip not protruding beyond the horizontal plane of the vertebral end-plate.

1. **Shear stresses across the disc** — more likely to be associated with a degenerative disc.

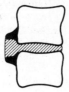

Lateral

Undulating Anterior Ossification
Undulating ossification of the anterior longitudinal ligament, intervertebral disc and paravertebral connective tissue.

1. **Diffuse idiopathic skeletal hyperostosis (DISH)**.

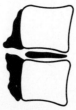

Lateral

2.14   Anterior Vertebral Body Beaks

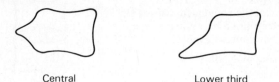

Central   Lower third

Involves 1–3 vertebral bodies at the thoracolumbar junction and usually associated with a kyphosis. Hypotonia is probably the common denominator which leads to an exaggerated thoracolumbar kyphosis, anterior herniation of the nucleus pulposus and subsequently an anterior vertebral body defect.

Central
1. **Morquio's syndrome***.

Lower Third
1. **Hurler's syndrome***.
2. **Achondroplasia***.
3. **Pseudoachondroplasia**.
4. **Cretinism***.
5. **Down's syndrome***.
6. **Neuromuscular diseases**.

Further Reading
Swischuk L.E. (1970) The beaked, notched or hooked vertebra. Its significance in infants and young children. *Radiology*, 95: 661–4.

2.15   Anterior Scalloping of Vertebral Bodies

1. **Aortic aneurysm** — intervertebral discs remain intact. Well-defined anterior vertebral margin. ± calcification in the wall of the aorta.
2. **Tuberculous spondylitis** — with marginal erosions of the affected vertebral bodies. Disc space destruction. Widening of the paraspinal soft tissues.
3. **Lymphadenopathy** — pressure resorption of bone results in a well-defined anterior vertebral body margin unless there is malignant infiltration of the bone.
4. **Delayed motor development** — e.g. Down's syndrome.

2.16   Anterior Scalloping of the Sacrum

1. **Metastases** (q.v.).
2. **Multiple myeloma***.
3. **Posterior soft tissue pelvic tumours** — invading bone or causing pressure resorption.
4. **Chordoma** — the majority of chordomas occur at this site. A bulky tumour. ± calcification.
5. **Anterior sacral meningocoele** — a round or oval defect in the anterior wall of the sacrum associated with a soft-tissue mass. The diagnosis is confirmed by myelography.

2.17   Posterior Scalloping of Vertebral Bodies

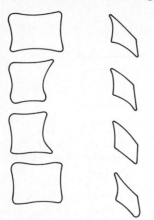

May be associated with
flattening of the pedicles
on the AP view

Scalloping is most prominent (a) at either end of the spinal canal,
(b) with large and slow growing lesions and (c) with those lesions
which originate during the period of active growth and bone
modelling.

1. **Tumours in the spinal canal** — ependymoma (especially of
   the filum terminale and conus), dermoid, lipoma, neurofibroma and less commonly meningioma.
2. **Neurofibromatosis*** — scalloping is due to a mesodermal
   dysplasia and is associated with dural ectasia. Localized
   scalloping can also result from pressure resorption by a
   neurofibroma, in which case there may also be enlargement of an intervertebral foramen and flattening of one
   pedicle ('dumb-bell tumour'). However, multiple wide
   thoracic intervertebral foramina are more likely due to
   lateral meningocoeles than to local tumours.
3. **Acromegaly*** — other spinal changes include increased AP
   and transverse diameters of the vertebral bodies giving a
   spurious impression of decreased vertebral height,
   osteoporosis, spur formation and calcified discs.
4. **Achondroplasia*** — with spinal stenosis and anterior
   vertebral body beaks.

5. **Communicating hydrocephalus** — if severe and untreated.
6. **Syringomyelia** — especially if the onset is before 30 years of age.
7. **Other congenital syndromes**
   (a) Ehlers–Danlos ⎱ both associated with dural ectasia.
   (b) Marfan's*. ⎰
   (c) Hurler's*.
   (d) Morquio's*.
   (e) Osteogenesis imperfecta tarda*.

Further Reading

Mitchell G.E., Lourie H. & Berne A.S. (1967) The various causes of scalloped vertebrae and notes on their pathogenesis. *Radiology*, 89: 67–74.

2.18   Widened Interpedicular Distance

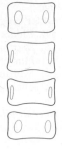

Most easily appreciated by comparison with
adjacent vertebrae. ± flattening of the inner side
of the pedicles.

1. **Meningomyelocoele** — fusiform distribution of widened
   interpedicular distances with the greatest separation at the
   midpoint of the involved segment. Disc spaces are
   narrowed and bodies appear to be widened. Spinous
   processes and laminae are not identifiable. Facets may be
   fused into a continuous mass. Scoliosis (congenital or
   developmental) in 50–70% of cases ± kyphosis.
2. **Intraspinal mass** (q.v.) — especially ependymoma.
3. **Diastematomyelia** — 50% occur between L1 and L3; 25%
   between T7 and T12. Widened interpedicular distances
   are common but not necessarily at the same level as the
   spur. The spur is visible in 33% of cases and extends from
   the neural arch forward. Laminar fusion associated with a
   neural arch defect at the same or adjacent level are
   important signs in predicting the presence of diastematomyelia. ± associated meningocoele, neurenteric cyst or
   dermoid.

2.19 Spinal Block

May be extradural, intradural or intramedullary.

1. **Widespread malignancy** — 42%.
2. **Neural tumours** — 20%.
3. **Disorders of intervertebral joints** — 15%.
4. **Primary bone disorders** — 13%.
5. **Arachnoiditis** — 6.5%.
6. **Others** — 4%.
   (a) Widespread infection.
   (b) Angioma.
   (c) Lipoma of cord.
   (d) Congenital cyst.
   (e) Spontaneous haemorrhage.

Further Reading
O'Carroll M.P. & Witcombe J.B. (1979) Primary disorders of bone with spinal block. *Clin. Radiol.*, 30: 299–306.

2.20   Extradural Spinal Masses

1. **Disc**— commonly lower cervical and
        lower lumbar. Rarely in thoracic
        region but even a small disc prot-
        rusion in this region may produce
        symptoms as the epidural space is
        smallest here. Congenital spinal
        stenosis may precipitate
        symptoms.

2. **Bone**
    (a) Osteophyte.
    (b) Metastases — breast and bronchus
        commonest. (NB disc destruction
        may occasionally occur in
        lymphoma and myeloma.)
    (c) Trauma — fracture or haematoma.
    (d) Paget's disease* — vertebral body enlarged with thick-
        ened cortex ('picture frame'). Neural arch may be
        involved. Paraspinal mass (osteoid tissue) may occur
        and may be calcified.
    (e) Osteomyelitis
        (i)   TB (disc destruction and calcified paraspinal
              mass).
        (ii) pyogenic.
        (iii) hydatid — extradural extension of disease in 30%
              of those with spinal involvement. In the early
              stages there is a well defined lucency in the
              vertebral body often extending into the pedicle,
              lamina or transverse process. Later there is ver-
              tebral body collapse.
    (f) Primary bone tumours
        (i)   Haemangioma* — due to compression fracture or
              chronic haemorrhage.
        (ii) Aneurysmal bone cyst*.
        (iii) Osteoblastoma*.
        (iv) Chordoma.

3. **Abscess** — commonly at the thoracolumbar junction. No
    bony abnormality if acute.

4. **Haematoma** — secondary to trauma or bleeding angioma.

5. **Arachnoid cyst** — commonly thoracic. Contains pulsatile
    CSF and scallops the posterior vertebra, flattens pedicles,
    and widens the interpedicular distance over several verteb-
    ral segments.

2.21 Intradural, Extramedullary Spinal Masses

1. **Neurofibroma** — any level. Bony erosion, expansion of the intervertebral foramina, splaying of ribs, posterior scalloping of vertebral body. Scoliosis in 40%. Paraspinal mass. No calcification. Equal sex incidence.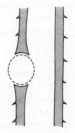
2. **Meningioma** — commonly thoracic. Only 10% show bony erosion and this is usually minimal. 90% occur on the lateral aspect of the dura. Can calcify, but difficult to see on X-ray. May cause paraspinal mass. 80% occur in females over 40.
3. **Lipoma** — commonly lower cervical/upper thoracic. Slow growth causes bony erosion. May extend over several vertebral segments. Associated with spinal dysraphism. Occurs in early adulthood.
4. **Dermoid** — commonly conus/cauda equina. Associated with spinal dysraphism.
5. **Angioma** — no bony abnormality.
6. **Ependymoma** — commonly filum terminale and so appears as an intradural mass. Can be enormous and cause bone erosion and expansion.
7. **Metastases from CNS tumour** — particularly medulloblastoma, glioblastoma, pinealoma and ependymoma.

2.22   Intradural, Intramedullary Spinal Masses

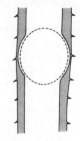

1. **Ependymoma** — commonest intramedullary spinal tumour. Usually conus,
   or filum terminale. Slow growth. Can be
   enormous and cause bone erosion and
   expansion.
2. **Glioma** — only slight bone erosion and
   expansion.
3. **Syringomyelia** — commonly no bony
   abnormality. 90% associated with
   Arnold–Chiari malformation. Occurs in
   early adulthood.
4. **Post-radiation myelopathy** — can cause symmetrical expansion of the cord which may extend beyond the irradiated
   segment, and may be indistinguishable from an intrinsic
   tumour.
5. **Haematoma** — due to contusion of the cord.

Bibliography

Allen E.H., Cosgrove D. & Millard F.J.C. (1978) The radiological
   changes in infections of the spine and their diagnostic value.
   Clin. Radiol., 29: 31–40.
Epstein B. (1976) *The Spine: A Radiological Text and Atlas*, 4th edn.
   Philadelphia: Lea & Febiger.
Felson B. (ed.) (1972) The spinal canal. *Semin. Roentgenol.*, 7(3).
Felson B. (ed.) (1979) Localised diseases of the spinal column. *Semin.
   Roentgenol.*, 14(1).
Lewtas N. (1980) The spine and myelography. In: Sutton D. (ed.)
   Textbook of Radiology and Imaging, 3rd edn. Edinburgh:
   Churchill Livingstone.
Sandrock A.R. (ed.) (1977) The spine. *Radiol. Clin. North Am.*,
   15(2).

Chapter 3
Joints

3.1 Monoarthritis

1. **Trauma** — pointers to the diagnosis are (a) the history, (b) the presence of a fracture and (c) a joint effusion, especially a lipohaemarthrosis.
2. **Osteoarthritis**.
3. **Crystal induced arthritis**
   (a) Gout*.
   (b) Calcium pyrophosphate dihydrate deposition disease*.
   (c) Calcium hydroxyapatite deposition disease.
4. **Rheumatoid arthritis*** — occasionally. Also juvenile chronic arthritis.
5. **Pyogenic arthritis** — commonest joints affected are the hip, knee and small joints of the hands and feet. 15% of those due to *Staphylococcus aureus* and 80% of those of gonococcal aetiology involve two or more joints. The joint may be radiologically normal at first clinical examination. Initially there is soft-tissue swelling due to effusion and synovial enlargement. Periarticular erosions progress to involve all of the articular cartilage and subchondral bone. Periosteal reaction. Osteoporosis follows the destructive changes.
6. **Tuberculous arthritis** — sometimes associated with pulmonary or renal tuberculosis. Similar sites of predilection to pyogenic arthritis. Insidious onset with radiological changes present at the time of first examination. Slowly developing osteoporosis precedes the destructive changes. Erosions first develop at peripheral non-contact points of the joint.
7. **Pigmented villonodular synovitis** — most commonly at the knee.
8. **Sympathetic** — a joint effusion can occur as a response to a tumour in the adjacent bone.

65

3.2   The Major Polyarthritides

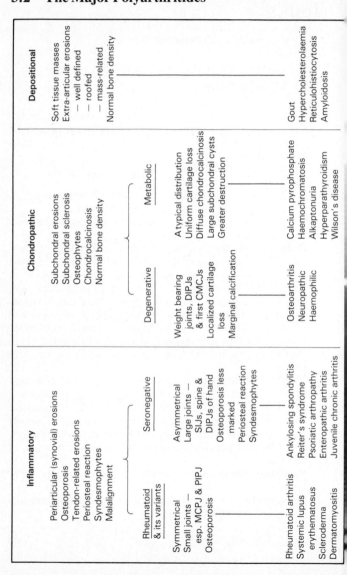

Inflammatory		Chondropathic		Depositional
Rheumatoid & its variants	**Seronegative**	**Degenerative**	**Metabolic**	
Periarticular (synovial) erosions	Asymmetrical	Subchondral erosions		Soft tissue masses
Osteoporosis	Large joints —	Subchondral sclerosis		Extra-articular erosions
Tendon-related erosions	SIJs, spine &	Osteophytes		— well defined
Periosteal reaction	DIPJs of hand	Chondrocalcinosis		— roofed
Syndesmophytes	Osteoporosis less	Normal bone density		— mass-related
Malalignment	marked			Normal bone density
	Periosteal reaction			
	Syndesmophytes			
		Weight bearing	A typical distribution	
Symmetrical		joints, DIPJs	Uniform cartilage loss	
Small joints —		& first CMCJs	Diffuse chondrocalcinosis	
esp. MCPJ & PIPJ		Localized cartilage	Large subchondral cysts	
Osteoporosis		loss	Greater destruction	
		Marginal calcification		
Rheumatoid arthritis	Ankylosing spondylitis	Osteoarthritis	Calcium pyrophosphate	Gout
Systemic lupus	Reiter's syndrome	Neuropathic	Haemochromatosis	Hypercholesterolaemia
erythematosus	Psoriatic arthropathy	Haemophilic	Alkaptonuria	Reticulohistiocytosis
Scleroderma	Enteropathic arthritis		Hyperparathyroidism	Amyloidosis
Dermatomyositis	Juvenile chronic arthritis		Wilson's disease	

3.3 Arthritis with Osteoporosis

1. **Rheumatoid arthritis***.
2. **Systemic lupus erythematosus***.
3. **Pyogenic arthritis**.
4. **Reiter's syndrome*** — in the acute phase.
5. **Scleroderma***.
6. **Haemophilia***.

3.4 Arthritis with Preservation of Bone Density

1. **Osteoarthritis**.
2. **Calcium pyrophosphate arthropathy** — see Calcium pyrophosphate dihydrate deposition disease*.
3. **Gout***.
4. **Psoriatic arthropathy***.
5. **Ankylosing spondylitis**.
6. **Reiter's syndrome*** — in chronic or recurrent disease.
7. **Neuropathic arthropathy*** — especially in the spine and lower extremities.
8. **Pigmented villonodular synovitis**.

3.5 Arthritis with a Periosteal Reaction

1. **Juvenile chronic arthritis***.
2. **Reiter's syndrome***.
3. **Pyogenic arthritis**.
4. **Psoriatic arthropathy***.
5. **Rheumatoid arthritis*** — in less than 5% of patients.
6. **Haemophilia***.

3.6   Arthritis with Preserved or Widened Joint Space

1. **Early infective or inflammatory arthritis** — because of joint effusion.
2. **Psoriatic arthropathy*** — due to deposition of fibrous tissue.
3. **Acromegaly*** — due to cartilage overgrowth.
4. **Gout***.
5. **Pigmented villonodular synovitis**.

3.7   Arthritis Mutilans

A destructive arthritis of the hands and feet with resorption of bone ends and telescoping joints (main-en-lorgnette).

1. **Rheumatoid arthritis***.
2. **Juvenile chronic arthritis***.
3. **Psoriatic arthropathy***.
4. **Diabetes**.
5. **Leprosy**.
6. **Neuropathic arthropathy***.
7. **Reiter's syndrome*** — in the feet.

3.8   Diffuse Terminal Phalangeal Sclerosis

1. **Normal variant**.
2. **Rheumatoid arthritis***.
3. **Scleroderma***.
4. **Systemic lupus erythematosus***.
5. **Sarcoidosis***.

3.9 Erosion (Enlargement) of the Intercondylar Notch of the Distal Femur

1. **Juvenile chronic arthritis*.**
2. **Haemophilia*.**
3. **Psoriatic arthropathy*.**
4. **Tuberculous arthritis.**
5. **Rheumatoid arthritis*.**

3.10 Calcified Loose Body (Single or Multiple) in a Joint

1. **Detached osteophyte** — larger and more variable in size than synovial osteochondromata. Other signs of degenerative arthritis.
2. **Osteochondral fracture.**
3. **Osteochondritis dissecans** — most commonly the knee, talus and elbow. A corresponding defect in the parent bone may be visible.
4. **Neuropathic arthropathy*** — joint disorganization.
5. **Synovial osteochondromatosis** — knee most commonly; hip, ankle, wrist and shoulder less commonly. Multiple small nodules of fairly uniform size. Faintly calcified initially; later ossified. Secondary erosion of intracapsular bone, joint space narrowing and osteophyte formation may occur later in the disease.

3.11 Calcification of Articular (Hyaline) Cartilage (Chondrocalcinosis)

1. **Calcium pyrophosphate dihydrate deposition disease*.**
2. **Hyperparathyroidism*.**
3. **Haemochromatosis*.**
4. **Acromegaly***
5. **Gout*.**
6. **Wilson's disease.**

3.12   Sacroiliitis

1. Changes initially in the lower and middle thirds of the joint and the iliac side is more severely affected than the sacral side.
2. Periarticular osteoporosis, superficial erosions and sclerosis of subchondral bone.
3. Further erosion leads to widening of the joint space.
4. Subchondral sclerosis progresses to bony ankylosis.
5. Eventual return of the bones to normal density.

The most typical patterns of distribution are:

Bilateral Symmetrical
1. **Ankylosing spondylitis*** — may be asymmetrical early in the disease. Radiological signs as above.
2. **Inflammatory bowel disease** — ulcerative colitis, Crohn's disease and Whipple's disease. Identical appearances to ankylosing spondylitis.
3. **Psoriatic arthropathy*** — ankylosis is less frequent than in ankylosing spondylitis. Occurs in 30–50% of patients with arthropathy. Less commonly is asymmetrical or unilateral.
4. **Osteitis condensans ilii** — predominantly in young, multiparous women. A triangular segment of bone sclerosis on the inferior aspect of the iliac side of the joint is associated with a well-defined joint margin and a normal joint space.
5. **Hyperparathyroidism*** — subchondral bone resorption and joint-space widening only.
6. **Paraplegia** — joint-space narrowing and osteoporosis.

Bilateral Asymmetrical
1. **Reiter's syndrome***.
2. **Psoriatic arthropathy*** — this pattern in 40% of cases.
3. **Rheumatoid arthritis*** — rare. Minimal sclerosis and no significant bony ankylosis.
4. **Gouty arthritis** (see Gout*) — large well-defined erosions with surrounding sclerosis.
5. **Osteoarthritis** — the articular margins are smooth and well defined. Joint-space narrowing, subchondral sclerosis and anterior osteophytes are observed.

Unilateral
1. **Infection**.

3.13 Protrusio Acetabuli

1. **Rheumatoid arthritis*** — including juvenile chronic arthritis.
2. **Osteoporosis** (q.v.).
3. **Osteomalacia and rickets** (q.v.)*.
4. **Paget's disease***.
5. **Ankylosing spondylitis***.
6. **Osteoarthritis** — occasionally.
7. **Trauma** — acetabular fractures.
8. **Familial or idiopathic**.

3.14 Widening of the Symphysis Pubis

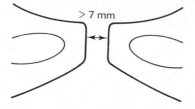

1. **Pregnancy** — a normal finding which can be accentuated by the patient standing on one leg.
2. **Trauma**.
3. **Osteitis pubis** — one or more months following parturition or pelvic surgery, especially prostatic surgery. It may also be observed as a chronic stress reaction in athletes. Symmetrical bone resorption with subchondral bony irregularity and sclerosis. Ankylosis may be a late finding.
4. **Ectopia vesicae**.
5. **Cleidocranial dysplasia*** — due to delayed or absent ossification.
6. **Infection** — low-grade osteomyelitis shows similar radiological features to osteitis pubis.
7. **Hyperparathyroidism*** — due to subperiosteal erosions.

3.15   Fusion or Bridging of the Symphysis Pubis

1. **Post-traumatic**.
2. **Post-infective**.
3. **Osteitis pubis** — see section 3.14.
4. **Osteoarthritis**.
5. **Ankylosing spondylitis***.
6. **Alkaptonuria***.
7. **Fluorosis**.

Bibliography

Forrester D.M., Brown J.C. & Nesson J.W. (1979) *The Radiology of Joint Disease*, 2nd edn. Philadelphia: Saunders.
Resnick D. & Niwayama G. (1981) *Diagnosis of Bone and Joint Disorders*. Philadelphia: Saunders.

Chapter 4
Respiratory Tract

4.1 Acute Upper Airway Obstruction

Most commonly in infants, because of the small calibre of the airways. Small or normal volume lungs with distension of the upper airway proximal to the obstruction during inspiration.

1. **Laryngo-tracheobronchitis** — narrowing of the glottic and subglottic regions. Indistinct tracheal margin because of oedema.
2. **Acute epiglottitis** — the epiglottis is swollen and may be shortened. Other components of the supraglottic region — aryepiglottic folds, arytenoids, uvula and prevertebral soft tissues — are also swollen. The hypopharynx and pyriform sinuses are distended with air.
3. **Retropharyngeal abscess** — enlargement of the prevertebral soft tissues which may contain gas or an air–fluid level.
4. **Oedema** — due to angio-oedema (allergic, anaphylactic or hereditary), inhalation of noxious gases or trauma. Predominantly laryngeal oedema.
5. **Foreign body** — more commonly produces a major bronchial occlusion rather than upper airway obstruction.
6. **Retropharyngeal haemorrhage** — due to trauma, neck surgery, direct carotid arteriography and bleeding disorders. Widening of the retropharyngeal soft-tissue space.

4.2   Chronic Upper Airway Obstruction in a Child

May be associated with overinflation of the lungs.

Supraglottic
1. **Laryngomalacia (congenital laryngeal stridor)** — presents shortly after birth, getting worse until 3–6 months, thereafter improving until it has resolved by 2 years. No specific radiological signs.
2. **Grossly enlarged tonsils and adenoids**.
3. **Micrognathia** — in the Pierre Robin syndrome.
4. **Cysts** — of the epiglottis or aryepiglottic folds. The degree of obstruction depends on the size and location.

Glottic
1. **Laryngeal polyp, papilloma or cyst**.

Subglottic and Tracheal
1. **Respiratory papillomatosis** — occur anywhere from the nose to the lungs. Irregular soft-tissue masses around the glottis or in the trachea mostly. (Papillomas in adults are usually single.)
2. **Subglottic haemangioma** — occurs before 6 months. Characteristically, it produces an asymmetrical narrowing of the subglottic region on the AP view.
3. **Tracheomalacia** — due to absent or defective cartilage rings. ± laryngomalacia and cleft palate. Dilated airway during inspiration and premature collapse during expiration.
4. **Following prolonged tracheal intubation** — see section 4.3.
5. **Vascular rings** — double aortic arch or an anomalous left subclavian artery. The trachea is displaced to the right and bowed anteriorly. Diagnosis is confirmed by aortography. See section 6.10.
6. **Anomalous origin of the left pulmonary artery from the right pulmonary artery** — which compresses the right main bronchus or lower trachea as it passes between the trachea and oesophagus to reach the left hilum.
7. **External compression from other mediastinal structures** —e.g. lymph nodes or an enlarged thymus.

Further Reading
Kushner, D.C. & Clifton Harris, G.B. (1978) Obstructing lesions of the larynx and trachea in infants and children. *Radiol. Clin. North Am.*, 16: 181–94.

4.3 Chronic Upper Airway Obstruction in an Adult

May be associated with overinflation of the lungs.

Supraglottic
1. **Supraglottic carcinoma of the larynx** — involving the posterior surface of the epiglottis, the ventricle or the superolateral part of the vestibule. Dyspnoea is a late feature.

Glottic
1. **Vocal cord paralysis** — airway obstruction is most likely with bilateral recurrent nerve paresis and this most commonly occurs as a result of thyroidectomy or malignant disease in the neck.
2. **Carcinoma of the glottis** — accounts for more than two-thirds of laryngeal carcinomas. Occurs mostly in the anterior two-thirds of the cords. Morphologically it can be proliferative or infiltrative.

Subglottic and Tracheal
1. **Extrinsic compression** — due to lymph nodes or local invasion from carcinomas of the bronchus, thyroid or oesophagus.
2. **Following prolonged tracheal intubation** — occurs in 5% of cases. The stenosis occurs most commonly at the level of the stoma. Less common sites are at the level of the inflatable cuff and where the tip impinged on the mucosa.
3. **Infraglottic carcinoma of the larynx** — either arising de novo at this site or as an extension from a glottic growth.
4. **Tracheal malignancy** — squamous cell carcinoma is the commonest tracheal primary.

Further Reading
Weber A.L. (ed.) (1978) The larynx and trachea. *Radiol. Clin. North Am.*, 16(2).

4.4   Unilateral Hypertransradiant Hemithorax

Exclude *contralateral* increased density, e.g. pleural effusion in a supine patient or pleural thickening.

Rotation
1. **Poor technique** ⎫ the hypertransradiant hemithorax is the
2. **Scoliosis** ⎭ side to which the patient is turned.

Chest Wall
1. **Mastectomy** — absent breast ± absent pectoral muscle shadows.
2. **Poliomyelitis** — atrophy of pectoral muscles ± atrophic changes in the shoulder girdle and humerus.
3. **Poland's syndrome** — unilateral congenital absence of pectoral muscles ± rib defects. Occurs in 10% of patients with syndactyly.

Pleura
1. **Pneumothorax** — note the lung edge and absent vessels peripherally.

Lung
1. **Compensatory emphysema** — following lobectomy (rib defects and opaque bronchial sutures indicate previous surgery) or lobar collapse.
2. **Obstructive emphysema** — due to bronchial stenosis or occlusion (q.v.). Air trapping on expiration results in increased lung volume and shift of the mediastinum to the contralateral side.
3. **Unilateral bullae** — vessels are absent rather than attenuated. May mimic pneumothorax.
4. **Macleod's syndrome** — the late sequela of childhood bronchiolitis. Small lung with small main and peripheral arteries. Air trapping occurs on expiration. Decreased number of bronchial divisions (5–10).

5. **Congenital lobar emphysema** — one-third present at birth. Marked overinflation of a lobe, most commonly the left upper lobe, right upper lobe or right middle lobe. The ipsilateral lobes are compressed and there is mediastinal displacement to the contralateral side.

Pulmonary Vessels
1. **Pulmonary embolus** (see Pulmonary embolic disease*) — to a major pulmonary artery (at least lobar in size). The pulmonary artery is dilated proximally and the affected lung shows moderate loss of volume.

4.5 Bilateral Hypertransradiant Hemithoraces

With Overexpansion of the Lungs

1. **Chronic obstructive emphysema** — with large central pulmonary arteries and peripheral arterial pruning. ± bullae.
2. **Asthma** — overinflation is secondary to bronchial constriction and mucus plugs.
3. **Acute bronchiolitis** — particularly affects children in the first year of life. Overexpansion is due to bronchial obstruction secondary to mucosal swelling and this produces bronchial wall thickening on the radiograph. Collapse or consolidation are not a primary feature of the condition but are frequent complications of it.
4. **Tracheal, laryngeal or bilateral bronchial stenoses** (q.v.).

With Normal or Small Lungs

1. **Congenital heart disease producing oligaemia** — includes those conditions with right heart obstruction and right-to-left shunts. The hila are usually small except when there is post-stenotic dilatation of the pulmonary artery.
2. **Pulmonary artery stenosis** — if due to valvar stenosis there will be post-stenotic dilatation. 60% of congenital lesions have other associated cardiovascular abnormalities.
3. **Multiple pulmonary emboli**
4. **Primary pulmonary hypertension**
5. **Schistosomiasis**
6. **Metastatic trophoblastic tumour**

{ identical radiological picture of big hilar vessels with peripheral pruning. History is most important. PPH occurs predominantly in young females and may be familial. Schistosomiasis more usually presents as a diffuse reticulonodular pattern.

Further Reading

Hodson M.E., Simon G. & Batten J.C. (1974) Radiology of uncomplicated asthma. *Thorax*, 29: 296–303.
Thurlbeck W.M. & Simon G. (1978) Radiographic appearance of the chest in emphysema. *Am. J. Roentgenol.*, 130: 427–40.

4.6 Bronchial Stenosis or Occlusion

In the Lumen
1. **Foreign body** — air trapping is more common than atelectasis. The lower lobe is most frequently affected. The foreign body may be opaque.
2. **Mucus plug** — in asthma or cystic fibrosis.
3. **Misplaced endotracheal tube**.
4. **Aspergillosis** — with thickened bronchial walls.

In the Wall
1. **Carcinoma of the bronchus** — tapered narrowing ± irregularity.
2. **Bronchial adenoma** — usually a smooth, rounded filling defect, convex toward the hilum.
3. **Sarcoid granuloma**.
4. **Fibrosis** — e.g. tuberculosis and fungi. Can mimic carcinoma but usually produces a longer constriction.
5. **Bronchial atresia** — most commonly the apico-posterior segment of the left upper lobe.
6. **Fractured bronchus**.

Outside the Wall
1. **Lymph nodes**
2. **Mediastinal tumour** ⎤
3. **Enlarged left atrium** ⎬ smooth, eccentric narrowing.
4. **Aortic aneurysm** ⎦
5. **Anomalous origin of left pulmonary artery from right pulmonary artery** — producing compression of the right main bronchus as it passes over it, between the trachea and oesophagus to reach the left hilum. PA chest X-ray shows the right side of the trachea to be indented and the vessel is seen end-on between the trachea and oesophagus on the lateral view.

4.7   Increased Density of a Hemithorax

With Central Mediastinum

1. **Consolidation** — ± air bronchogram. Includes pneumonia, unilateral oedema (q.v.), aspiration pneumonia and radiation pneumonitis.
2. **Pleural effusion** — when the patient is supine a small or moderate effusion gravitates posteriorly producing a generalized increased density with an apical cap of fluid. Erect or decubitus films confirm the diagnosis.
3. **Mesothelioma** — often associated with a pleural effusion which obscures the tumour. Encasement of the lung limits mediastinal shift. ± pleural calcification.

With Mediastinal Displacement away from the Dense Hemithorax

1. **Pleural effusion** (q.v.) — N.B. a large effusion with no mediastinal shift implies underlying collapse which, in an older person, is often secondary to a bronchial carcinoma.
2. **Diaphragmatic hernia** — on the right side with herniated liver; on the left side the hemithorax is not usually opaque because of air within the herniated bowel. The left hemithorax may be opaque in the early neonatal period when air has not yet had time to reach the herniated bowel.

With Mediastinal Displacement towards the Dense Hemithorax

1. **Collapse**.
2. **Post-pneumonectomy** — rib resection ± opaque bronchial sutures.
3. **Lymphangitis carcinomatosa** — unilateral disease is uncommon. Linear and nodular opacities ± ipsilateral hilar and mediastinal lymphadenopathy. Septal lines.
4. **Pulmonary agenesis and hypoplasia** — usually asymptomatic. Absent or hypoplastic pulmonary artery.

N.B. 70% of unilateral diffuse *lung* opacities involve the right lung. Pneumonia, aspiration, pulmonary oedema, lymphangitis carcinomatosa and radiotherapy account for 90% (Youngberg 1977).

Further Reading

Youngberg A.S. (1977) Unilateral diffuse lung opacity. *Radiology*, 123: 277–82.

4.8 Pneumatocoeles

One or more air-filled, thin-walled 'cysts'. They are usually infective in origin and are thought to result from a check valve obstruction of a communication between a cavity and a bronchus. They appear during the first two weeks of the pneumonia and resolve within several months. They may contain fluid levels.

Infections
1. *Staphylococcus aureus* — a characteristic feature of childhood staphylococcal pneumonia, developing in 40–60% of cases.
2. *Streptococcus pneumoniae*.
3. *Escherichia coli*.
4. *Klebsiella pneumoniae*.
5. *Haemophilus influenzae*.
6. *Legionella pneumophila* (**Legionnaire's disease**).

Traumatic
1. **Interstitial emphysema** — may be followed by thin-walled air-containing cysts.

4.9 Slowly Resolving or Recurrent Pneumonia

1. **Bronchial obstruction** (q.v.) — especially neoplasm or foreign body.
2. **Inappropriate chemotherapy** — especially for tuberculosis, Klebsiella and mycoses.
3. **Repeated aspiration**
   (a) Pharyngeal pouch.
   (b) Achalasia.
   (c) Scleroderma*.
   (d) Hiatus hernia.
   (e) 'H'-type tracheo-oesophageal fistula.
   (f) Paralytic or neuromuscular disorders.
   (g) Chronic sinusitis.
4. **Underlying lung pathology**
   (a) Abscess.
   (b) Bronchiectasis — see section 4.13.
   (c) Cystic fibrosis*.

5. **Immunological incompetence**
    (a) Cachexia.
    (b) Steroids and immunosuppressives.
    (c) Diabetes.
    (d) White-cell and immunoglobulin deficiency states.
6. **Pneumonias that resolve by fibrosis**
    (a) Tuberculosis.
    (b) Fungi.

4.10   Pneumonia with an Enlarged Hilum

Hilar lymph-node enlargement may be secondary to the pneumonia or pneumonia may be secondary to bronchial obstruction by a hilar mass. Signs suggestive of a secondary pneumonia are:
(a) Segmental or lobar consolidation which is better defined than a primary pneumonia.
(b) Slow resolution.
(c) Recurrent consolidation in the same part of the lung.
(d) Associated collapse.

Secondary Pneumonias
See section 4.6, but note particularly 'Carcinoma of the bronchus'.

Primary Pneumonias
1. **Primary tuberculosis** — lymph-node enlargement is unilateral in 80% and involves the hilar (60%), or combined hilar and paratracheal (40%) nodes.
2. **Viral pneumonias** — especially pertussis.
3. **Mycoplasma** — lymph-node enlargement is common in children but rare in adults. May be uni- or bilateral.
4. **Primary histoplasmosis** — in endemic areas. Hilar lymphadenopathy is common, particularly in children. During healing the lymph nodes calcify and may cause bronchial obstruction thereby initiating distal infection.
5. **Coccidioidomycosis** — in endemic areas. The pneumonic type consists of predominantly lower lobe consolidation which is frequently associated with hilar lymph-node enlargement.

See also section 4.29.

4.11   Lobar Pneumonia

Consolidation involving the air spaces of an anatomically recognizable lobe. The entire lobe may not be involved and there may be a degree of associated collapse.

1. *Streptococcus pneumoniae* — the commonest cause. Usually unilobar. Cavitation rare. Pleural effusion is uncommon. Little or no collapse.
2. *Klebsiella pneumoniae* — often multilobar involvement. Great propensity for cavitation and lobar enlargement.
3. *Staphylococcus aureus* — especially in children. 40–60% of children develop pneumatocoeles. Effusion (empyema) and pneumothorax are also common. Bronchopleural fistula may develop. No lobar predilection.
4. **Tuberculosis** — in primary or post-primary tuberculosis, but more common in the former. Associated collapse is common. The right lung is affected twice as often as the left and primary tuberculosis predilects the anterior segment of the upper lobe or the medial segment of the middle lobe.
5. *Streptococcus pyogenes* — affects the lower lobes predominantly. Often associated with a pleural effusion.

4.12   Consolidation with Lobar Enlargement

Homogeneous or inhomogeneous air space opacification with bulging of the bounding fissures.

1. *Klebsiella pneumoniae* — lobar enlargement occurs before cavitation.
2. **Abscess** — when an area of consolidation breaks down. Organisms which commonly produce abscesses are *Staphylococcus aureus*, *Klebsiella* spp. and other Gram-negative organisms.
3. **Carcinoma of the bronchus** — this can fill and expand a lobe but is usually not contained by the fissures.

4.13   Bronchiectasis

1. Peribronchial thickening and retained secretions.
2. Crowded vessels, i.e. loss of volume.
3. Compensatory emphysema.
4. Cystic spaces ± air fluid levels.
5. Coarse honeycomb pattern in very severe disease.
6. Normal radiograph in 7%.

1. **Secondary to childhood infections** — especially measles and pertussis.
2. **Secondary to bronchial obstruction** — foreign body, neoplasm, mucus plugs (cystic fibrosis and asthma) and aspergillosis.
3. **Chronic aspiration**.
4. **Congenital structural defects**
   (a) Kartagener's syndrome — bronchiectasis with immobile cilia, dextro cardia and absent frontal sinuses. 5% of patients with dextrocardia will eventually develop bronchiectasis.
   (b) Williams–Campbell syndrome — bronchial cartilage deficiency.
5. **Immune deficiency states** — e.g. hypogammaglobulinaemia, chronic granulomatous disease and Chédiak–Higashi syndrome.

4.14   Widespread Alveolar Opacities

1. Early appearance after onset of symptoms.
2. Ill-defined margins.
3. Early coalescence.
4. Air bronchogram and air alveologram.
5. Rapid change.

1. **Oedema** (q.v.).
2. **Pneumonia** — most often the unusual types
   (a) Tuberculosis.
   (b) Histoplasmosis.
   (c) Pneumocystis carinii.
   (d) Influenza — particularly in patients with mitral stenosis or who are pregnant.
   (e) Chicken pox — may be confluent in the central areas of the lungs. ± hilar lymph-node enlargement.
   (f) Other viral pneumonias.
3. **Haemorrhage**
   (a) Trauma (contusion).
   (b) Anticoagulants, haemophilia, leukaemia and disseminated intravascular coagulopathy.
   (c) Goodpasture's syndrome.
   (d) Idiopathic pulmonary haemosiderosis — in the acute stage.
4. **Fat emboli** — 1–2 days post-trauma. Predominantly peripheral. Resolves in 1–4 weeks.
5. **Alveolar cell carcinoma** — effusions are common. Mediastinal lymph nodes are uncommon. Diagnosis by sputum cytology or lung biopsy.
6. **Haematogenous metastases** — especially chorioncarcinoma. Others are rare.
7. **Lymphoma*** — usually with hilar or mediastinal lymphadenopathy.
8. **Sarcoidosis*** — often associated with a reticulonodular pattern elsewhere.
9. **Löffler's** — peripheral ('reversed bat's wing'), often in the upper zones.

4.15 Localized Alveolar Opacities

See 'Widespread alveolar opacities', section 4.14.

1. **Pneumonia**.
2. **Infarction** (see Pulmonary embolic disease*) — usually in the lower lobes. Often indistinguishable from pneumonia.
3. **Contusion** — ± rib fractures or other signs of trauma.
4. **Oedema** (q.v.).
5. **Radiation** — several weeks following radiotherapy. May have a straight margin, corresponding to the field of treatment.
6. **Alveolar cell carcinoma**.
7. **Lymphoma***.

4.16   Pulmonary Oedema

1. **Heart failure**.
2. **Fluid overload** — excess i.v. fluids, renal failure and excess hypertonic fluids, e.g. contrast media.
3. **Cerebral disease** — cerebrovascular accident, head injury or raised intracranial pressure.
4. **Near drowning** — radiologically no significant differences between fresh-water and sea-water drowning.
5. **Aspiration (Mendelson's syndrome)**.
6. **Radiotherapy** — several weeks following treatment. May have a characteristic straight edge.
7. **Rapid re-expansion of lung following thoracentesis**.
8. **Liver disease and other causes of hypoproteinaemia**.
9. **Transfusion reaction**.
10. **Drugs**
    (a) Those which induce cardiac arrhythmias or depress myocardial contractility.
    (b) Those which alter pulmonary capillary wall permeability, e.g. overdoses of heroin, morphine, methadone, dextropropoxyphene and aspirin. Hydrochlorothiazide, phenylbutazone, aspirin and nitrofurantoin can cause oedema as an idiosyncratic response.
    N.B. Contrast media can induce arrhythmias, alter capillary wall permeability and produce a hyperosmolar load.
11. **Poisons**
    (a) Inhaled — NO_2, SO_2, CO, Phosgene, hydrocarbons and smoke.
    (b) Circulating — Paraquat and snake venom.
12. **Mediastinal tumours** — producing venous or lymphatic obstruction.
13. **Shock lung (adult respiratory distress syndrome)** — 24–72 hours post insult.

4.17   Unilateral Pulmonary Oedema

Pulmonary Oedema on the Same Side as a Pre-existing Abnormality

1. **Prolonged lateral decubitus position**.
2. **Unilateral aspiration**.
3. **Pulmonary contusion**.
4. **Rapid thoracentesis of air or fluid**.
5. **Bronchial obstruction**.
6. **Systemic artery to pulmonary artery shunts** — e.g. Waterston (on the right side), Blalock–Taussig (left or right side) and Pott's procedure (on the left side).

Pulmonary Oedema on the Opposite Side to a Pre-existing Abnormality

i.e. oedema on the side opposite a lung with a perfusion defect.

1. **Congenital absence or hypoplasia of a pulmonary artery**.
2. **Macleod's syndrome**.
3. **Thromboembolism.**
4. **Unilateral emphysema**.
5. **Lobectomy**.
6. **Pleural disease**.

Further Reading

Calenoff L., Kruglik G.D. & Woodruff A. (1978) Unilateral pulmonary oedema. *Radiology*, 126: 19–24.

4.18   Septal Lines (Kerley B Lines)

1. Due to visible interlobular lymphatics and their surrounding connective tissue.
2. 1–3 cm long, less than 1 mm thick, extending from and perpendicular to the pleural surface.
3. Best seen in the costophrenic angles.

Pulmonary Venous Hypertension

1. **Left ventricular failure**.
2. **Mitral stenosis**.

Lymphatic Obstruction

1. **Pneumoconioses** — surrounding tissues may contain a heavy metal, e.g. tin, which contributes to the density.
2. **Lymphangitis carcinomatosa**.
3. **Sarcoidosis*** — septal lines are uncommon.

4.19 'Honeycomb Lung'

1. A generalized reticular pattern or miliary mottling which when summated produces the appearance of air containing 'cysts' 0.5–2.0 cm in diameter.
2. Obscured pulmonary vasculature.
3. Late appearance of radiological signs after the onset of symptoms.
4. Complications
   (a) pneumothorax is frequent;
   (b) cor pulmonale later in the course of the disease.

1. **Collagen disorders**
   (a) Rheumatoid lung — most pronounced at the bases and may be preceded by basal infiltrates. ± small effusions.
   (b) Scleroderma* — predominantly basal. Less regular 'honeycomb' pattern, which is preceded by fine, linear, basal streaks. Cor pulmonale is unusual.
2. **Extrinsic allergic alveolitis*** — predominantly in the upper zones.
3. **Sarcoidosis*** — sparing of extreme apices. Hilar lymphadenopathy usually resolved by this stage but if present it is a useful sign.
4. **Pneumoconiosis** — particularly frequent in asbestosis*, but also in other reactive dusts.
5. **Cystic bronchiectasis** (q.v.) — in lower and middle lobes especially. Bronchial-wall thickening. ± localized areas of consolidation.
6. **Cystic fibrosis***.
7. **Drugs** — nitrofurantoin, busulphan, cyclophosphamide, bleomycin and melphalan.
8. **Histiocytosis X*** — 'honeycomb' pattern probably always preceded by disseminated nodules. May be predominantly in the mid and upper zones. Cor pulmonale is uncommon.
9. **Tuberous sclerosis*** — lung involvement in 5% of patients. Symptoms first in adult life. Differentiated clinically.
10. **Idiopathic interstitial fibrosis (cryptogenic fibrosing alveolitis)** — no specific differentiating features. More marked in the lower half of the lungs initially and progresses to involve the whole of the lungs.
11. **Neurofibromatosis*** — ± rib notching, 'ribbon' ribs and/or scoliosis. In 10%, but not before adulthood.

4.20   Pneumoconioses

Inorganic Dusts

WITHOUT FIBROSIS
1. **Ferric oxide** — siderosis.
2. **Ferric oxide + silver** — argyrosiderosis.
3. **Tin oxide** — stannosis.
4. **Barium** — barytosis.
5. **Calcium**.

WITH FIBROSIS
1. **Free silica** — silicosis*.
2. **Coal dust** — coal miner's pneumoconiosis*.
3. **Silicates** — asbestosis*, china clay, talc and mica.

WITH CHEMICAL PNEUMONITIS
1. **Beryllium**.
2. **Manganese**.
3. **Vanadium**.
4. **Osmium**.
5. **Cadmium**.

CARCINOGENIC DUSTS
1. **Radioactive dusts** — e.g. uranium.
2. **Asbestos** — see Asbestosis*.
3. **Arsenic**.

Organic Dusts (Extrinsic Allergic Alveolitis*)
1. **Mouldy hay** — farmers' lung.
2. **Bagasse (sugar cane dust)** — bagassosis.
3. **Cotton or linen dust** — byssinosis.
4. **Mouldy vegetable compost** — mushroom worker's lung.
5. **Pigeon and budgerigar excreta** — pigeon breeder's and budgerigar fancier's lung.

Further Reading

Felson B (ed.) (1967) The pneumoconioses. *Semin. Roentgenol.*, 2 (3).
Fraser R.G. & Pare J.A.P. (1975) Extrinsic allergic alveolitis. *Semin. Roentgenol.*, 10: 31–42.

4.21   Multiple Pin-point Opacities

Must be of very high atomic number to be rendered visible.

1. **Post lymphogram** — iodized oil emboli. Contrast medium may be visible at the site of termination of the thoracic duct.
2. **Silicosis*** — usually larger than pin-point but can be very dense, especially in goldminers.
3. **Stannosis** — inhalation of tin oxide. Even distribution throughout the lungs. With Kerley A and B lines.
4. **Barytosis** — inhalation of barytes. Very dense, discrete opacities. Generalized distribution but bases and apices usually spared.
5. **Limestone and marble workers** — inhalation of calcium.
6. **Alveolar microlithiasis** — familial. Lung detail obscured by miliary calcifications. Few symptoms but may progress to cor pulmonale eventually. Pleura, heart and diaphragm may be seen as negative shadows.

4.22   Multiple Opacities (0.5–2 mm)

Soft-tissue Density
1. **Miliary tuberculosis** — widespread. Uniform size. Indistinct margins but discrete. No septal lines. Normal hila unless superimposed on primary tuberculosis.
2. **Fungal diseases** — miliary histoplasmosis, coccidioidomycosis, blastomycosis and cryptococcosis (torulosis). Similar appearance to miliary tuberculosis.
3. **Coal miner's pneumoconiosis*** — predominantly mid zones with sparing of the extreme bases and apices. Ill defined and may be arranged in a circle or rosette. Septal lines.
4. **Sarcoidosis*** — predominantly mid zones. Ill defined. Often with enlarged hila.
5. **Acute extrinsic allergic alveolitis*** — micronodulation in all zones, but predominantly basal.
6. **Fibrosing alveolitis** — initially most prominent in the lower halves of the lungs and later spreads upwards. Poorly defined. Obliteration of vascular markings.

Greater than Soft-tissue Density

1. **Haemosiderosis** — secondary to chronic raised venous pressure (seen in 10–15% of patients with mitral stenosis), repeated pulmonary haemorrhage (e.g. Goodpasture's disease) or idiopathic. Septal lines. Smaller than miliary TB.
2. **Silicosis*** — relative sparing of bases and apices. Very well defined and dense when due to pure silica; ill defined and of lower density when due to mixed dusts. Septal lines.
3. **Siderosis** — lower density than silica. Widely disseminated. Asymptomatic.
4. **Stannosis** ⎱ see section 4.21.
5. **Barytosis** ⎰

4.23 Multiple Opacities (2–5 mm)

Remaining Discrete

1. **Carcinomatosis** — breast, thyroid, sarcoma, melanoma, prostate, pancreas or bronchus (eroding a pulmonary artery). Variable sizes and progressive increase in size. ± lymphatic obstruction.
2. **Lymphoma*** — nearly always with hilar or mediastinal lymphadenopathy.
3. **Sarcoidosis*** — predominantly mid zones. Often with enlarged hila.

Tending to Confluence and Varying Rapidly

1. **Multifocal pneumonia** — including aspiration pneumonia and tuberculosis.
2. **Pulmonary oedema** (q.v.).
3. **Extrinsic allergic alveolitis*** — predominantly basal.
4. **Fat emboli** — predominantly peripheral.

4.24 Solitary Pulmonary Nodule

Granulomas

1. *Tuberculoma* — more common in the upper lobes and on the right side. Well defined. 0.5–4 cm. 25% are lobulated. Calcification frequent. 80% have satellite lesions. Cavitation is uncommon and when present is small and eccentric. Usually persist unchanged for years.
2. **Histoplasmoma** — in endemic areas (Mississippi and the Atlantic coast of USA). More frequent in the lower lobes. Well defined. Seldom larger than 3 cm. Calcification is common and may be central producing a target appearance. Cavitation is rare. Satellite lesions are common.

Malignant Neoplasms

1. **Carcinoma of the bronchus** — usually greater than 2 cm. Accounts for less than 15% of all solitary nodules at 40 years; almost 100% at 80 years. Appearances suggesting malignancy are
   (a) Recent appearance or rapid growth (previous CXRs are very helpful here).
   (b) Size greater than 4 cm.
   (c) The lesion crosses a fissure (although some fungus diseases also do so).
   (d) Ill-defined margins.
   (e) Umbilicated or notched margin (if present it indicates malignancy in 80%).
   (f) Corona radiata (spiculation). (But also seen in PMF and granulomas.)
   (g) Peripheral line shadows.
   (h) Calcification is very rare, except in scar carcinomas.
2. **Metastasis** — accounts for 3–5% of asymptomatic nodules. 25% of pulmonary metastases are solitary. Most likely primaries are breast, sarcoma, seminoma and renal cell carcinoma. Predilection for the lung periphery. Calcification is rare but occurs with metastatic osteosarcoma, chondrosarcoma and some other rarer metastases.
3. **Alveolar cell carcinoma** — when localized, a mass is the most common presentation. More commonly ill defined. Air bronchogram is common. No calcification. Pleural effusion in 5%. Mediastinal lymphadenopathy is much less common than with carcinoma of the bronchus.

Benign Neoplasms
1. **Adenoma** — 90% occur around the hilum; 10% are peripheral. Round or oval and well defined. 25% present as a solitary nodule; 75% present with the effects of bronchial stenosis. Calcification and cavitation are rare. Histologically, 80–90% are carcinoids and 10–20% are cylindromas. The former may metastasize to bone (sclerotic secondaries) or to liver and may produce the carcinoid syndrome.
2. **Hamartoma** — 96% occur over 40 years. 90% are intrapulmonary and usually within 2 cm of the pleura. 10% produce bronchial stenosis. Usually less than 4 cm diameter. Well defined. Lobulated rather than smooth. Calcification in 30%, although the incidence increases with the size of the lesion (in 75% when greater than 5 cm). Calcification is 'popcorn', craggy or punctate.

Infections
1. **Pneumonia** — simple consolidation, especially pneumococcal. Air bronchogram.
2. **Hydatid** — in endemic areas. Most common in the lower lobes and more frequent on the right side. Well defined. 1–10 cm. Solitary in 70%. May have a bizarre shape. Rupture results in the 'water lily' sign.

Congenital
1. **Sequestration** — usually more than 6 cm. Two-thirds occur in the left lower lobe, one-third in the right lower lobe and contiguous to the diaphragm. Well defined, round or oval. Diagnosis confirmed by aortography and venous drainage is via the pulmonary veins (intralobar type) or bronchial veins (extralobar type).
2. **Bronchogenic cyst** — peak incidence in the 2nd and 3rd decades. Two-thirds are intrapulmonary and occur in the medial one-third of the lower lobes. Round or oval. Smooth walled and well defined.

Vascular
1. **Pulmonary infarction** (see Pulmonary embolic disease*) — most frequent in the lower lobes. With a pleural effusion and elevation of the hemidiaphragm.
2. **Haematoma** — peripheral, smooth and well defined. 2–6 cm. Slow resolution over several weeks.
3. **Arteriovenous malformation** — 66% are single. Well defined, lobulated ('bag of worms'). Tomography may show feeding or draining vessels. Calcification is rare.

4.25 Multiple Pulmonary Nodules (greater than 5 mm)

Neoplastic
1. **Metastases** — most commonly from breast, thyroid, kidney, gastrointestinal tract and testes. In children, Wilms' tumour, Ewing's tumour, neuroblastoma and osteosarcoma. Predilection for lower lobes and more common peripherally. Range of sizes. Well defined. Ill-definition suggests prostrate, breast or stomach. Hilar lymphadenopathy and effusions are uncommon.

Infections
1. **Abscesses** — widespread distribution but asymmetrical. Commonly *Staphylococcus aureus*. Cavitation common. No calcification.
2. **Coccidioidomycosis** — in endemic areas. Well defined with a predilection for the upper lobes. 0.5–3 cm. Calcification and cavitation may be present.
3. **Histoplasmosis** — in endemic areas. Round, well defined and few in number. Sometimes calcify. Usually unchanged for many years.
4. **Hydatid** — more common on the right side and in the lower zones. Well defined unless there is surrounding pneumonia. Often 10 cm or more. May rupture and show the 'water lily' sign.

Immunological

1. **Wegener's granulomatosis** — widespread distribution. 0.5–10 cm. Round and well defined. No calcification. Cavitation in 30–50% of cases. ± focal pneumonitis.
2. **Rheumatoid nodules** — peripheral and more common in the lower zones. Round and well defined. No calcification. Cavitation common.
3. **Caplan's syndrome** — well defined. Develop rapidly in crops. Calcification and cavitation occur. Background stippling of pneumoconiosis.

Inhalational

1. **Progressive massive fibrosis** — mid and upper zones. Begin peripherally and move centrally. Peripheral emphysema. Oval in shape. Calcification and cavitation occur. Background nodularity of pneumoconiosis.

Vascular

1. **Arteriovenous malformations** — 33% are multiple. Well defined. Lobulated. Tomography may show feeding or draining vessels. Calcification is rare.

4.26 Lung Cavities

Infective, i.e. Abscesses
1. **Staphylococcus aureus** — thick walled with a ragged inner lining. No lobar predilection. Associated with effusion and empyema ± pyopneumothorax — almost invariable in children, not so common in adults. Pneumatocoeles (q.v.). Multiple.
2. **Klebsiella pneumoniae** — thick walled with a ragged inner lining. More common in the upper lobes. Usually single but may be multilocular. ± effusion.
3. **Tuberculosis** — thick walled and smooth. Upper lobes and apical segment of lower lobes mainly. Usually surrounded by consolidation. ± fibrosis.
4. **Aspiration** — look for foreign body, e.g. tooth.
5. **Others** — Gram-negative organisms, actinomycosis, nocardiosis, histoplasmosis, coccidioidomycosis, aspergillosis, hydatid and amoebiasis.

Neoplastic
1. **Carcinoma of the bronchus** — thick walled with an eccentric cavity. Predilection for the upper lobes. Found in 2–10% of carcinomas and especially if peripheral. More common in squamous cell carcinomas and may then be thin walled.
2. **Metastases** — thin or thick walled. May only involve a few of the nodules. Seen especially in squamous cell, colon and sarcoma metastases.
3. **Hodgkin's disease** — thin or thick walled and typically in an area of infiltration. With hilar or mediastinal lymphadenopathy.

Vascular
1. **Infarction** — more common in the lower lobes. Thick walled with a shaggy inner lining. ± effusion and elevation of the hemidiaphragm.

Abnormal Lung
1. **Cystic bronchiectasis** (q.v.) — thin walled. More common in the lower lobes.
2. **Infected emphysematous bulla** — thin walled. ± air fluid level.
3. **Sequestrated lung** — thick or thin walled. 66% in the right lower lobe, 33% in the left lower lobe. ± air fluid level. ± surrounding pneumonia.
4. **Bronchogenic cyst** — in medial third of lower lobes. Thin walled. ± air fluid level. ± surrounding pneumonia.

Granulomas
1. **Wegener's granulomatosis** — widespread. Cavitation in some of the nodules. Thick walled, becoming thinner with time. Can be transient.
2. **Rheumatoid nodules** — thick walled with a smooth inner lining. Especially in the lower lobes and peripherally. Well defined. Become thin walled with time.
3. **Progressive massive fibrosis** — predominantly in the mid and upper zones. Thick walled and irregular. Background nodularity.

Traumatic
1. **Haematoma** — peripheral. Air fluid level if it communicates with a bronchus.
2. **Traumatic lung cyst** — thin walled and peripheral. Single or multiple. Uni- or multilocular. Distinguished from cavitating haematomas as they present early, within hours of the injury.

4.27   Opacity with an Air Bronchogram

Infective
1. **Pneumonia**.

Inflammatory
1. **Radiation pneumonitis**.
2. **Progressive massive fibrosis**.

Neoplastic
1. **Alveolar cell carcinoma**.
2. **Lymphoma***.
3. **Lymphosarcoma**.

4.28 Multiple Pulmonary Calcifications

1. **Infections**
   (a) Tuberculosis — primary or post-primary. Upper zone predominance.
   (b) Histoplasmosis — in endemic areas. Similar to tuberculosis but the calcifications may have a faint halo producing target lesions.
   (c) Coccidioidomycosis.
   (d) Chicken pox — following chicken pox pneumonia in adulthood. 1–3 mm. Numbered in 10s.
2. **Chronic pulmonary venous hypertension** — especially mitral stenosis. Most prominent in the mid and lower zones.
3. **Silicosis*** — in up to 20% of those showing nodular opacities.
4. **Caplan's syndrome**.
5. **Metastases** — especially osteogenic sarcoma and chondrosarcoma. Others include papillary carcinoma of the thyroid, cystadenocarcinoma of the ovary and mucinous adenocarcinomas of the gastrointestinal tract or breast.
6. **Lymphoma following radiotherapy**.
7. **Alveolar microlithiasis** — often familial. Myriad minute calcifications in alveoli which obscure all lung detail. Because of the lung's increased density, the heart, pleura and diaphragm may be evident as negative shadows.
8. **Metabolic** — in primary and secondary hyperparathyroidism, hypervitaminosis D and milk-alkali syndrome.

Further Reading

Maile C.W., Rodan B.A., Godwin J.D., Chen J.T.T. & Ravin C.E. (1982) Calcification in pulmonary metastases. *Br. J. Radiol.*, 55: 108–13.

4.29   Unilateral Hilar Enlargement

Lymph Nodes
1. **Carcinoma of the bronchus** — the hilar enlargement may be due to the tumour itself or involved lymph nodes.
2. **Lymphoma*** — unilateral is very unusual; involvement is usually bilateral and asymmetrical.
3. **Infective**
   (a) Primary tuberculosis.
   (b) Histoplasmosis.
   (c) Coccidioidomycosis.
   (d) Mycoplasma.
   (e) Pertussis.
4. **Sarcoidosis*** — unilateral disease in only 1–5%.

Pulmonary Artery
1. **Post-stenotic dilatation** — on the left side.
2. **Pulmonary embolus** (see Pulmonary embolic disease*) — massive to one lung. Peripheral oligaemia.
3. **Aneurysm** — in chronic pulmonary arterial hypertension. ± egg-shell calcification.

Others
1. **Mediastinal mass** (q.v.) — superimposed on a hilum.
2. **Perihilar pneumonia** — ill defined, ± air bronchogram.

See also section 4.10.

4.30   Bilateral Hilar Enlargement

Due to lymph node enlargement or pulmonary artery enlargement.

Idiopathic
1. **Sarcoidosis*** — symmetrical and lobulated. Bronchopulmonary ± unilateral or bilateral paratracheal lymphadenopathy.

Neoplastic
1. **Lymphoma*** — asymmetrical.
2. **Lymphangitis carcinomatosa**.

Infective
1. **Viruses** — most common in children.
2. **Primary tuberculosis** — rarely bilateral and symmetrical.
3. **Histoplasmosis**.
4. **Coccidioidomycosis**.

Vascular
1. **Pulmonary arterial hypertension** — see section 5.15.

Immunological
1. **Extrinsic allergic alveolitis*** — in mushroom workers.

Inhalational
1. **Silicosis*** — symmetrical.
2. **Chronic berylliosis** — only in a minority of cases. Symmetrical.

4.31 'Eggshell' Calcification of Lymph Nodes

Peripheral, rim calcification, predominantly involving the hilar lymph nodes.

1. **Silicosis*** — seen in approximately 5% of silicotics. Predominantly hilar lymph nodes but may also be observed in the anterior and posterior mediastinal lymph nodes, cervical lymph nodes and intraperitoneal lymph nodes. More frequently seen in complicated pneumoconiosis. Lungs show multiple small nodular shadows or areas of massive fibrosis.
2. **Sarcoidosis*** — calcification of lymph nodes occurs in approximately 5% of patients and is occasionally 'eggshell' in appearance. There may be extensive lymph-node involvement throughout the mediastinum. Calcification appears about 6 years after the onset of the disease and is almost invariably associated with advanced pulmonary disease and in some cases with steroid therapy. The pulmonary manifestations include reticulonodular, acinar or fibrotic changes in the mid to upper zones.
3. **Lymphoma following radiotherapy** — appears 1–9 years post radiotherapy.
4. **Coal miner's pneumoconiosis*** — occurs in only 1% of cases. Associated pulmonary changes include miliary shadowing or massive shadows.

Differential Diagnosis
1. **Pulmonary artery calcification** — a rare feature of pulmonary arterial hypertension.
2. **Aortic calcification** — especially in the wall of a saccular aneurysm.
3. **Anterior mediastinal tumours** — teratodermoids and thymomas may occasionally exhibit rim calcification.

4.32   Upper Zone Fibrosis

1. **Tuberculosis** — calcification frequent.
2. **Radiotherapy** — no calcification. ± evidence of the cause, e.g. mastectomy for carcinoma, or radiation osteonecrosis of ribs or clavicle.
3. **Sarcoidosis*** — no calcification. ± 'eggshell' calcification of lymph nodes.
4. **Chronic extrinsic allergic alveolitis***.
5. **Histoplasmosis** — similar to tuberculosis.
6. **Progressive massive fibrosis** — conglomerate infiltrates with peripheral emphysema. Background nodularity. ± 'eggshell' calcification of lymph nodes.
7. **Ankylosing spondylitis*** — resembles tuberculosis. Cavitation frequent with mycetoma. Disease is almost invariably bilateral and associated with severe spondylitis.

Further Reading

Howarth F.H., Kendall M.J., Lawrence D.S. & Whitfield A.G.W. (1975) Chest radiograph in ankylosing spondylitis. *Clin. Radiol.*, 26: 455–60.

4.33   Pleural Effusion

Transudate (protein < 30 gl^{-1})
1. **Cardiac failure**.
2. **Hepatic failure**.
3. **Nephrotic syndrome**.
4. **Meigs' syndrome**.

Exudate (protein > 30 gl^{-1})
1. **Infection**.
2. **Malignancy**.
3. **Pulmonary infarction** — see Pulmonary embolic disease*.
4. **Collagen vascular diseases**.
5. **Subphrenic abscess**.
6. **Pancreatitis**.

Haemorrhagic
1. **Carcinoma of the bronchus**.
2. **Trauma**.
3. **Pulmonary infarction** — see Pulmonary embolic disease*.
4. **Bleeding disorders**.

Chylous
1. **Obstructed thoracic duct** — due to trauma, malignant invasion or filariasis.

4.34   Pleural Effusion with an Otherwise Normal Chest X-ray

Effusion may be the only abnormality or other signs may be obscured by the effusion.

Infective
1. **Primary tuberculosis** — more common in adults (40%) than children (10%). Rarely bilateral.
2. **Viruses and mycoplasma** — effusions occur in 10–20% of cases but are usually small.

Neoplastic
1. **Carcinoma of the bronchus** — effusion occurs in 10% of patients and a peripheral carcinoma may be hidden by the effusion.
2. **Metastases** — most commonly from breast; less commonly pancreas, stomach, ovary and kidney.
3. **Mesothelioma** — effusion in 90%; often massive and obscures the underlying pleural disease.
4. **Lymphoma*** — effusion occurs in 30% but is usually associated with lymphadenopathy or pulmonary infiltrates.

Immunological
1. **Systemic lupus erythematosus*** — effusion is the sole manifestation in 10% of cases. Usually small but may be massive. Bilateral in 50%. 35–50% of those with an effusion have associated cardiomegaly.
2. **Rheumatoid disease** (see Rheumatoid arthritis*) — observed in 3% of patients. Almost exclusively males. Usually unilateral and may antedate joint disease. Tendency to remain unchanged for a long time.

Extrathoracic Diseases
See section 4.35.

Others

1. **Pulmonary embolus** (see Pulmonary embolic disease*) — effusion is a common sign and it may obscure an underlying area of infarction.
2. **Closed chest trauma** — effusion may contain blood, chyle or food (due to oesophageal rupture). The latter is almost always left-sided.
3. **Asbestosis*** — mesothelioma and carcinoma of the bronchus should be excluded but an effusion may be present without these complications. Effusion is frequently recurrent and usually bilateral. Usually associated with pulmonary disease.

4.35   Pleural Effusion due to Extrathoracic Disease

1. **Pancreatitis** — acute, chronic or relapsing. Effusions are predominatly left-sided. Elevated amylase content.
2. **Subphrenic abscess** — with elevation and restriction of movement of the ipsilateral diaphragm and basal atelectasis or consolidation.
3. **Following abdominal surgery** — most often seen on the side of the surgery and larger after upper abdominal surgery. Disappears after 2 weeks.
4. **Meigs syndrome** — pleural effusion + ascites + benign pelvic tumour (most commonly an ovarian fibroma, thecoma, granulosa cell tumour or cystadenoma).
5. **Nephrotic syndrome**.
6. **Fluid overload** — e.g. due to renal disease.
7. **Cirrhosis**.

4.36 Pneumothorax

1. **Spontaneous** — M:F, 8:1. Especially those of tall thin stature. ? due to ruptured blebs or bullae. 20% are associated with a small pleural effusion.
2. **Iatrogenic** — e.g. postoperative, after chest aspiration, during artificial ventilation, after lung biopsy or following attempted insertion of a subclavian venous line.
3. **Traumatic** — ± rib fractures, haemothorax, surgical emphysema or mediastinal emphysema.
4. **Secondary to mediastinal emphysema** (q.v.).
5. **Secondary to lung disease**
   (a) Emphysema.
   (b) 'Honeycomb lung' (q.v.).
   (c) Cystic fibrosis*.
   (d) Pneumonia.
   (e) Broncho-pleural fistula, e.g. due to lung abscess or carcinoma.
   (f) Lung neoplasms — especially metastases from osteogenic sarcomas and other sarcomas.
6. **Pneumoperitoneum** — air passes through a pleuro-peritoneal foramen.

4.37   Pneumomediastinum

May be associated with pneumothorax and subcutaneous emphysema.

1. **Lung tear** — a sudden rise in intra-alveolar pressure, often with airway narrowing, causes air to dissect through the interstitium to the hilum and then to the mediastinum.
    (a) Spontaneous — the most common cause and may follow coughing or strenuous exercise.
    (b) Asthma.
    (c) Diabetic ketoacidosis — related to severe and protracted vomiting.
    (d) Childbirth — because of repeated Valsalva manoeuvres.
    (e) Artificial ventilation.
    (f) Chest trauma.
2. **Perforation of oesophagus, trachea or bronchus** — ruptured oesophagus is often associated with a hydrothorax or hydropneumothorax, usually on the left side.
3. **Perforation of a hollow abdominal viscus** — with extension of gas via the retroperitoneal space.

Further Reading
Fraser R.G. & Paré J.A.P. (1979) Pneumomediastinum. In: Fraser R.G. & Paré J.A.P. (Eds) *Diagnosis of Diseases of the Chest*, 2nd edn, pp. 1810–17. Philadelphia: Saunders.

4.38 Unilateral Elevated Hemidiaphragm

Causes Above the Diaphragm
1. **Phrenic nerve palsy** — smooth hemidiaphragm. No movement on respiration. Paradoxical movement on sniffing. The mediastinum is usually central. The cause, e.g. bronchial carcinoma or mediastinal nodes, may be evident on the X-ray.
2. **Pulmonary collapse.**
3. **Pulmonary infarction** — see Pulmonary embolic disease*.
4. **Pleural disease** — especially old pleural disease, e.g. haemothorax, empyema or thoracotomy.
5. **Splinting of the diaphragm** — associated with rib fractures or pleurisy.
6. **Hemiplegia** — an upper motor neurone lesion.

Diaphragmatic Causes
1. **Eventration** — more common on the left side. The heart is frequently displaced to the contralateral side. Limited movement on normal respiration and paradoxical movement on sniffing. Stomach may show a partial volvulus.

Causes Below the Diaphragm
1. **Gaseous distension of the stomach or splenic flexure** — left hemidiaphragm only.
2. **Subphrenic inflammatory disease** — subphrenic abscess, hepatic or splenic abscess and pancreatitis.

Scoliosis
The raised hemidiaphragm is on the side of the concavity.

Decubitus Film
The raised hemidiaphragm is on the dependent side.

Differential Diagnosis
1. **Subpulmonary effusion** — movement of fluid is demonstrable on a decubitus film. On the left side there is increased distance between lung and stomach fundal gas.
2. **Ruptured diaphragm** — more common on the left. Barium meal confirms the diagnosis.

4.39   Bilateral Elevated Hemidiaphragms

Poor Inspiratory Effort

Obesity

Causes Above the Diaphragms
1. **Bilateral basal pulmonary collapse** — which may be secondary to infarction or subphrenic abscesses.
2. **Small lungs** — fibrotic lung disease, e.g. fibrosing alveolitis.

Causes Below the Diaphragms
1. **Ascites**.
2. **Pregnancy**.
3. **Pneumoperitoneum**.
4. **Hepatosplenomegaly**.
5. **Large intra-abdominal tumour**.
6. **Bilateral subphrenic abscesses**.

Differential Diagnosis
1. **Bilateral subpulmonary effusions**.

4.40   Pleural Calcification

1. **Old empyema**

2. **Old haemothorax**

Amorphous bizarre, plaques, often with a vacuolated appearance near the inner surface of greatly thickened pleura. Usually unilateral.

3. **Asbestos exposure** (see Asbestosis*) — small curvilinear plaques in the parietal pleura. More delicate than (1) and (2). Often multiple and bilateral and found over the domes of the diaphragms and immediately deep to the ribs. Observed in 50% of people exposed to asbestos but not before 20 years have elapsed. Not necessarily associated with asbestosis, i.e. pulmonary disease.
4. **Silicosis***
5. **Talc exposure**

similar appearances to asbestos exposure.

4.41   Local Pleural Masses

1. **Loculated pleural effusion**.
2. **Metastases** — from bronchus or breast. Often multiple.
3. **Malignant mesothelioma** — nearly always due to asbestos exposure. Extensive thickening of the pleura which may be partly obscured by an effusion. Little mediastinal shift. Adjacent bone destruction in 12%.
4. **Pleural fibroma (local benign mesothelioma)** — a smooth lobular mass, 2–15 cm diameter, arising more frequently from the visceral pleura than the parietal pleura. Tendency to change position with respiration as 30–50% are pedunculated. They form an obtuse angle with the chest wall which indicates their extrapulmonary location. Usually found in patients over 40 years of age and usually asymptomatic. However it causes hypertrophic osteoarthropathy in a greater proportion of cases than any other disease.
5. **Fibrin balls** — develop in a serofibrinous pleural effusion and become visible following absorption of the fluid. They are small and tend to be situated near the lung base. They may disappear spontaneously or remain unchanged for many years.

Differential Diagnosis
1. **Extrapleural masses** — see section 4.42.
2. **Plombage** — the insertion of foreign material into the extrapleural space as a treatment for tuberculosis. The commonest materials used were solid Lucite spheres, hollow 'ping-pong' balls (which may have fluid levels in them) or crumpled cellophane. They produce a well-defined, smooth pleural surface, convex inferiorly and medially and displacing the lung apex. The pleura makes an acute angle with the chest wall.

4.42   Rib Lesion with an Adjacent Soft-tissue Mass

Neoplastic
1. **Bronchogenic carcinoma** — solitary site unless metastatic.
2. **Metastases** — solitary or multiple.
3. **Multiple myeloma*** — classically multiple sites and bilateral.
4. **Mesothelioma** — rib destruction occurs in 12%.
5. **Lymphoma***.
6. **Fibrosarcoma** — similar appearances to mesothelioma.
7. **Neurofibroma** — rib notching.

Infective
1. **Tuberculous osteitis** — commonest inflammatory lesion of a rib. Second only to malignancy as a cause of rib destruction. Clearly defined margins ± abscess.
2. **Actinomycosis** ⎫ usually a single rib. Adjacent consoli-
3. **Nocardiosis** ⎭ dation.
4. **Blastomycosis** — adjacent patchy or massive consolidation ± hilar lymphadenopathy.

Inflammatory
1. **Radiation osteitis**.

Metabolic
1. **Renal osteodystrophy** ⎫ rib fractures and osteopenia
2. **Cushing's syndrome** ⎬ associated with a subpleural ⎭ haematoma.

Further Reading
Steiner R.M., Cooper M.W. & Brodovsky H. (1982) Rib destruction: a neglected finding in malignant mesothelioma. *Clin. Radiol.*, 33: 61–5.

4.43 The Chest Radiograph Following Chest Trauma

Soft Tissues
1. **Foreign bodies**.
2. **Surgical emphysema**.

Ribs
1. **Simple fracture** ⎫
2. **Flail chest** ⎬ may be associated with surgical emphysema, pneumothorax, extra-pleural haematoma or haemothorax. First-rib fractures have a high incidence of other associated injuries.

Sternum
1. **Fracture** — may be associated with an unsuspected dorsal spine fracture.

Clavicles
1. **Fracture**.

Spine
1. **Fracture**.
2. **Cord trauma**.
3. **Nerve root trauma** — especially to the brachial plexus.

Pleura
1. **Pneumothorax** — simple or tension.
2. **Haemothorax**.

Lung
1. **Contusion** — non-segmental alveolar opacities. Resolve in a few days.
2. **Haematoma** — usually appears following resolution of contusion. Round, well-defined nodule. Resolution in several weeks.
3. **Aspiration pneumonitis**.
4. **Foreign bodies**.
5. **Pulmonary oedema** — following blast injuries.
6. **Adult respiratory distress syndrome** — widespread alveolar shadowing appearing 24–72 hours after injury.
7. **Fat embolism**.

Trachea and Bronchi

1. **Laceration or fracture** — initially surgical emphysema and pneumomediastinum followed by collapse of the affected lung or lobe.

Diaphragm

1. **Rupture** — 90% occur on the left side. ± herniation of stomach or colon.

Mediastinum

1. **Aortic dissection** — widening of the mediastinum, blurring of the aortic shadow, apical effusion, tracheal shift and depression of the left main bronchus.
2. **Traumatic aortic aneurysm** — usually saccular.
3. **Mediastinal haematoma** — blurring of the mediastinal outline.
4. **Mediastinal emphysema** (q.v.).
5. **Haemopericardium**.
6. **Oesophageal rupture**.

Further Reading

Dow J., Roebuck E.J. & Cole F. (1970) Dissecting aneurysms of the aorta. *Br. J. Radiol.*, 39: 915–27.

Joffe N. (1974) The adult respiratory distress syndrome. *Am. J. Roentgenol.*, 122: 719–32.

Reynolds J. & Davis J.T. (1966) Thoracic injuries. The radiology of trauma. *Radiol. Clin. North Am.*, 4: 383–402.

4.44   Neonatal Respiratory Distress

Pulmonary Causes

A. WITH NO MEDIASTINAL SHIFT

1. **Hyaline membrane disease** — in premature infants. Fine granular pattern throughout both lungs, air bronchograms and, later, obscured heart and diaphragmatic outlines. Often cardiomegaly. May progress to a complete 'white-out'. Interstitial emphysema, pneumomediastinum and pneumothorax are frequent complications of ventilator therapy.

2. **Transient tachypnoea of the newborn** — prominent interstitial markings and vessels, thickened septa, small effusions and mild cardiomegaly. Resolves within 24 hours.

3. **Meconium aspiration syndrome** — predominatly post-mature infants. Coarse linear and irregular opacities of uneven size, generalized hyperinflation and focal areas of collapse and emphysema. Spontaneous pneumothorax and effusions in 20%. No air bronchograms.

4. **Pneumonia** — segmental or lobar consolidation. May resemble hyaline membrane disease or meconium aspiration syndrome, but should be suspected if unevenly distributed.

5. **Pulmonary haemorrhage** — 75% are less than 2.5 kg. Onset at birth or delayed several days. Resembles meconium aspiration syndrome or hyaline membrane disease.

6. **Upper airway obstruction** — e.g. choanal atresia and micrognathia.

7. **Mikity–Wilson syndrome (pulmonary dysmaturity)** — always premature infants and usually less than 1.5 kg. Initially well but there is an insidious onset of respiratory distress between 1 and 6 weeks. Streaky opacities radiating from both hila with small bubbly areas of focal hyper-aeration throughout both lungs. Moderate hyperinflation. Severe disease leads to death but infants may recover fully. Resolution over a period of 12 months. Bases clear before apices and hyperinflation is the last feature to disappear.

8. **Abnormal thoracic cage** — e.g. osteogenesis imperfecta and Jeune's thoracic dysplasia.

B. WITH MEDIASTINAL SHIFT AWAY FROM THE ABNORMAL SIDE

1. **Diaphragmatic hernia** — 6× more common on the left side. Multiple lucencies due to gas containing bowel in the chest. Herniated bowel may appear solid if X-rayed too early but there will still be a paucity of gas in the abdomen.
2. **Congenital lobar emphysema** — involves the left upper, right upper and right middle lobes (in decreasing order of frequency) with compression of the lung base (cf. pneumothorax which produces symmetrical lung compression).
3. **Cystic adenomatoid malformation** — translucencies of various shapes and sizes scattered throughout an area of opaque lung with well-defined margins.
4. **Pleural effusion (empyema, chylothorax)** — rare.

C. WITH MEDIASTINAL SHIFT TOWARDS THE ABNORMAL SIDE

1. **Atelectasis** — most commonly due to incorrect placement of an endotracheal tube down a major bronchus. Much less commonly primary atelectasis may occur without any other abnormality.
2. **Agenesis** — rare. May be difficult to differentiate from collapse but other congenital defects especially hemivertebrae are commonly associated.

Cardiac Causes (q.v.).

Cerebral Causes
Haemorrhage, oedema and drugs. After cardiopulmonary causes these account for 50% of the remainder.

Metabolic Causes
Metabolic acidosis, hypoglycaemia and hypothermia.

Abdominal Causes
Massive organomegaly, e.g. polycystic kidneys, elevating the diaphragms.

4.45   Ring Shadows in a Child

Neonate
1. **Diaphragmatic hernia** — unilateral.
2. **Interstitial emphysema** — secondary to ventilator therapy. Bilateral.
3. **Cystic adenomatoid malformation** — unilateral.
4. **Mikity–Wilson syndrome** — bilateral.

Older Child
1. **Cystic bronchiectasis** (q.v.).
2. **Cystic fibrosis***.
3. **Pneumatocoeles** (q.v.).
4. **Histiocytosis X*** ⎫   see 'Honeycomb lung', section
5. **Neurofibromatosis*** ⎭   4.19.

See also section 4.44.

4.46   Drug-induced Lung Disease

Lung Parenchyma
1. **Diffuse pneumonitis** — methotrexate, procarbazine and azathioprine.
2. **Diffuse pneumonitis progressing to fibrosis** — nitrofurantoin, melphalan, busulphan, cyclophosphamide and bleomycin.
3. **Pneumonitis associated with drug-induced systemic lupus erythematosus** — procainamide, hydralazine and isoniazid.
4. **Pulmonary haemorrhage** — anticoagulants and those drugs which produce an idiosyncratic thrombocytopenia.
5. **Pulmonary eosinophilia** — sulphonamides, chlorpropamide, sulphasalazine and imipramine.
6. **Allergic alveolitis** — pituitary snuff.

Pulmonary Vasculature
1. **Pulmonary oedema**
   (a) Excess intravenous fluids.
   (b) Altered capillary wall permeability — heroin, dextro-propoxyphene, methyldopa, hydrochlorothiazide, aspirin, nitrofurantoin and contrast media.
   (c) Drug-induced cardiac arrhythmias or impaired myocardial contractility.
2. **Pulmonary emboli** — high oestrogen oral contraceptives causing thromboemboli and oily emboli following lymph-angiography.

Bronchospasm
1. **β-blockers**.
2. **Histamine liberators** — iodine containing contrast media and morphine.
3. **Drugs as antigens** — antisera, penicillins and cephalospor-ins.
4. **Others** — aspirin, anti-inflammatory agents, paracetamol.

Hilar Enlargement or Mediastinal Widening
Phenytoin and steroids.

Increased Opportunistic Infections
1. **Antimitotics**.
2. **Steroids**.
3. **Actinomycin C**.
4. **Drug-induced neutropenia or aplastic anaemia** — idio-syncratic or dose-related.

Further Reading
Millar J.W. (1982) Drugs and the lungs. *Medicine International*, 1(20): 944–7.
Morrison D.A. & Goldman A.L. (1979) Radiographic patterns of drug induced lung disease. *Radiology*, 131: 299–304.

4.47 Anterior Mediastinal Masses

Anterior to the pericardium and trachea. Superiorly the retrosternal air space is obliterated. For ease of discussion it can be divided into three regions:

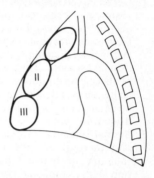

Region I

1. **Retrosternal goitre** — goitre extends into the mediastinum in 1–3% of cases. On a PA chest X-ray it appears as an inverted truncated cone with its base uppermost. It is well defined, smooth or lobulated. The trachea may be displaced posteriorly and laterally and may be narrowed. Calcification is common. Uptake by ^{131}I is diagnostic when positive but they are seldom functioning.
2. **Tortuous innominate artery** — a common finding in the elderly.
3. **Lymph nodes** — due to reticuloses, metastases or granulomas.
4. **Thymic masses** — the normal thymus is visible in 50% of neonates. On the PA view it is sail-shaped and more prominent on the right side. It is also more prominent in expiration, on a lordotic view and with oblique projections. An enlarged thymus in a child can be due to hyperparathyroidism, leukaemia, lymphoma, histiocytosis X or progeria.
   Thymic tumours are uncommon but occur in 20% of patients with myasthenia gravis. They are round or oval and smooth or lobulated. They may contain nodular or rim calcification. If it contains a large amount of fat (thymolipoma) then it may be very large and soft and reach the diaphragm, leaving the superior mediastinum clear.
5. **Aneurysm of the ascending aorta.**

Region II
1. **Germinal cell neoplasms** — including dermoids, teratomas, seminomas, choriocarcinomas, embryonal carcinomas and endodermal sinus tumours. More than 80% are benign and they occur with equal incidence to thymic tumours. Usually larger than thymomas (but not thymolipomas). Round or oval and smooth. They usually project to one or other side of the mediastinum on the PA view. Calcification, especially rim calcification, and fragments of bone or teeth may be demonstrable, the latter being diagnostic.
2. **Thymic tumours** — see Thymic masses (above).
3. **Sternal tumours** — metastases (breast, bronchus, kidney and thyroid) are the most common. Of the primary tumours, malignant (chondrosarcoma, myeloma, reticulum cell sarcoma and lymphoma) are more common than benign (chondroma, aneurysmal bone cyst and giant cell tumour).

Region III (Anterior Cardiophrenic Angle Masses)
1. **Pericardiac fat pad** — especially in obese people. A triangular opacity in the cardiophrenic angle on the PA view. It appears less dense than expected because of the fat content. CT is diagnostic. Excessive mediastinal fat can be due to steroid therapy.
2. **Diaphragmatic hump** — or localized eventration. Commonest on the anteromedial portion of the right hemidiaphragm. A portion of liver extends into it and this can be confirmed by ultrasound or isotope examination of the liver.
3. **Morgagni hernia** — through the defect between the septum transversum and the costal portion of the diaphragm. It is almost invariably on the right side but is occasionally bilateral. It usually contains a knuckle of colon or, less commonly, colon and stomach. Appears solid if it contains only omentum. Barium studies will confirm the diagnosis.
4. **Pericardial cysts** — either a true pericardial cyst ('spring water' cyst) or a pericardial diverticulum. The cyst is usually situated in the right cardiophrenic angle and is oval or spherical. CT confirms the liquid nature of the mass.

4.48 Middle Mediastinal Masses

Between the anterior and posterior mediastinum and containing the heart, great vessels and pulmonary roots. Causes of cardiac enlargement are excluded.

1. **Lymph nodes** — the paratracheal, tracheobronchial, bronchopulmonary and/or subcarinal nodes may be enlarged. This may be due to neoplasm (most frequently metastatic bronchial carcinoma), reticuloses (most frequently Hodgkin's disease), infection (most commonly tuberculosis, histoplasmosis or coccidioidomycosis) or sarcoidosis.
2. **Carcinoma of the bronchus** — arising from a major bronchus.
3. **Aneurysm of the aorta** — CT scanning after i.v. contrast medium or, if this is not available, aortography is diagnostic. Peripheral rim calcification is a useful sign if present.
4. **Bronchogenic cyst** — usually close to the carina and related to one of the major bronchi. Smooth, non-lobulated and well defined it projects above one or other hila on the PA chest X-ray. Usually posterior to the trachea on the lateral projection. No calcification. Rarely it communicates with the bronchial tree and will then contain a cavity.

4.49   Posterior Mediastinal Masses

Posterior to the posterior pericardial surface. For ease of
discussion it can be divided
into three regions:

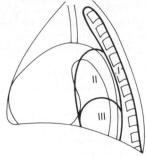

Region I (Paravertebral)

1. **Neurogenic tumours** — usually benign and more frequent in
   children and young adults. All the different tumour types
   look very similar: well defined, round or oval and smooth,
   lying in the paravertebral region. Ganglioneuromas are
   said to have a broader base towards the mediastinum.
   Calcification is rare but more common in malignant
   tumours. Benign tumours may cause pressure erosion of
   adjacent vertebral bodies, transverse processes or ribs;
   malignant tumours produce irregular bone destruction.
2. **Other paravertebral masses** (q.v.) — usually elongated
   and bilateral.
   (a) Abscess — with disc space and vertebral body
       destruction.
   (b) Extramedullary haemopoiesis — with splenomegaly
       ± bone changes of specific disease entities, e.g.
       haemolytic anaemias.
   (c) Reticuloses, myeloma and metastases — bone des-
       truction with preserved discs.
3. **Anterior thoracic meningocoele** — mainly in patients with
   neurofibromatosis. A well-defined mass anterior to the
   spine which projects laterally into the lung fields. The spine
   shows hemivertebra, 'butterfly' vertebra or other congenital abnormalities. The diagnosis is confirmed by myelography in the prone position.

Region II
1. **Dilated oesophagus** — especially achalasia. Contains mottled gas shadows ± an air fluid level. Diagnosis is confirmed by barium swallow.
2. **Aortic aneurysm** — the diagnosis is confirmed by arteriography.
3. **Neuroenteric cyst** — oval with a vertical long axis. It is closely related to the oesophagus which is usually displaced or indented. If it contains neural elements then there are associated congenital vertebral abnormalities.

Region III
1. **Hiatus hernia** — often contains an air fluid level which is projected through the cardiac shadow on a penetrated PA view.
2. **Bochdalek hernia** — through a persistent pleuroperitoneal canal. The contents may be stomach, colon, liver, spleen or kidney.

Bibliography

General

Felson B. (1973) *Chest Roentgenology*. Philadelphia: Saunders.
Fraser R.G. & Pare J.A.P. (1979) *Diagnosis of Diseases of the Chest*, 2nd edn. Philadelphia: Saunders.
Simon G. (1978) *Principles of Chest X-Ray Diagnosis*, 4th edn. London: Butterworths.
Sutton D. (ed.) (1980) *Textbook of Radiology and Imaging*, 3rd edn, chaps 11–21. Edinburgh: Churchill Livingstone.

Diffuse Pulmonary Disease, Emphysema and Pneumoconiosis

Crofton J. (1978) Diffuse pulmonary abnormalities: clinical correlations. *Clin. Radiol.*, 29: 353–62.
Cunningham C.D.B. & Hugh A.E. (1973) Pneumoconiosis in women. *Clin. Radiol.*, 24: 491–3.
Felson B. (ed.) (1967) The pneumoconioses. *Semin. Roentgenol.*, 2(3).
Felson B. (1979) A new look at pattern recognition of diffuse pulmonary disease. *Am. J. Roentgenol.*, 133: 183–9.
Fraser R.G. (1974) The radiologist and obstructive airway disease. *Am. J. Roentgenol.*, 120: 737–75.
Thurlbeck W.M. & Simon G. (1978) Radiographic appearance of the chest in emphysema. *Am. J. Roentgenol.*, 130: 427–40.

Infections

Balikian J.P. & Mudarris F.F. (1974) Hydatid disease of the lungs. A roentgenological study of 50 cases. *Am. J. Roentgenol.*, 122: 692–707.
Connell J. V. & Muhim J.R. (1976) Radiographic manifestations of pulmonary histoplasmosis. *Radiology*, 121: 281–5.
Felson B. (ed.) (1970) Fungus diseases of the lungs. *Semin. Roentgenol.*, 5(1).
Felson B. (ed.) (1979) Thoracic tuberculosis. *Semin. Roentgenol.*, 16(3).
Felson B. (ed.) (1980) The acute pneumonias. *Semin. Roentgenol.*, 15(1).
Felson B. (ed.) (1980) Lobar collapse. *Semin. Roentgenol.*, 15(2).
Forrest J.V. & Potchen E.J. (eds) (1973) Radiology of the chest. *Radiol. Clin. North Am.*, 11(1).
Freundlich I.M. & Israel H.L. (1973) Pulmonary aspergillosis. *Clin. Radiol.*, 24: 246–53.
Gordonson J., Birnbaum W., Jacobson G. & Sargent E.N. (1974) Pulmonary cryptococcosis. *Radiology*, 112: 557–61.
Klein D.L. & Gamsu G. (1980) Thoracic manifestations of aspergillosis. *Am. J. Roentgenol.*, 134: 543–52.
Vaněk J. & Schwarz J. (1971) The gamut of histoplasmosis. *Am. J. Med.*, 50: 89–104.

Neoplasms

Bateson E.M. (1964) The solitary bronchogenic carcinoma, 100 cases. *Br. J. Radiol.*, 37: 598–607.
Felson B. (ed.) (1977) Pulmonary neoplasms. *Semin. Roentgenol.*, 12(3).
Grainger R.G. (1975) Benign tumours of the respiratory tract. Clinical presentation and radiological features. In: Lant A.F. (ed.) Eleventh Symposium of Advanced Medicine, pp. 353–63. London: Royal College of Physicians.
Higgins G.A., Shields T.W. & Keehn R.J. (1975) The solitary pulmonary nodule. Ten year follow-up V.A.S.A.G. study. *Arch. Surg.*, 110: 570–5.
Libshitz H.I. & North L.B. (1982) Pulmonary metastases. *Radiol. Clin. North Am.*, 20(3), 437–51.
Rigler L.G. (1955) The roentgen signs of carcinoma of the lung. *Am. J. Roentgenol.*, 74: 415–28.

Miscellaneous

Fataar S. & Schulman A. (1979) Diagnosis of diaphragmatic tears. *Br. J. Radiol.*, 52: 375–81.
Felson B. (ed.) (1975) Immunology and the lung. *Semin. Roentgenol.*, 10(1).
Goodman L.R. (1980) Post-operative chest radiograph: I. Alterations after abdominal surgery. *Am. J. Roentgenol.*, 134: 533–41.
Goodman L.R. (1980) Post-operative chest radiograph: II. Alterations after major intrathoracic surgery. *Am. J. Roentgenol.*, 134: 803–13.
Joffe N. (1974) The adult respiratory distress syndrome. *Am. J. Roentgenol.*, 122: 719–32.
McGregor M.B.B. & Sandler G. (1964) Wegener's granulomatosis. *Br. J. Radiol.*, 37: 430–9.

Chapter 5
Cardiovascular System

5.1 Gross Cardiac Enlargement

1. **Multiple valvular disease** — aortic and mitral valve disease, particularly with regurgitation.
2. **Pericardial effusion** — no recognizable chamber enlargement. Flask-shaped heart on the erect film which becomes globular on the supine film. Acute angle between right heart border and right hemidiaphragm. The effusion masks ventricular wall movement; therefore, unusually sharp cardiac outline on the chest radiograph and poor pulsation on fluoroscopy. Rapid change in size on serial films. Diagnosis best made by echocardiography.
3. **ASD** — with pulmonary pleonaemia or an Eisenmenger situation.
4. **Cardiomyopathy** — including ischaemia.
5. **Ebstein's anomaly** — the posterior or septal cusp of the tricuspid valve arises distally from the wall of the right ventricle. Marked tricuspid incompetence. Marked right atrioventricular enlargement. Small aorta. Oligaemic lungs. Sharp cardiac outline.

5.2 Small Heart

1. **Normal variant**.
2. **Emphysema**.
3. **Addison's disease**.
4. **Dehydration/malnutrition**.
5. **Constrictive pericarditis**.

5.3 Enlarged Right Atrium

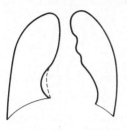

PA
Prominent right heart
border

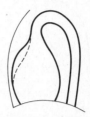

Lateral
Prominent anterosuperior
part of cardiac shadow

Volume Overload
1. **ASD**.
2. **AV canal**.
3. **Tricuspid incompetence** — including Ebstein's anomaly, endocardial fibroelastosis and endomyocardial fibrosis.
4. **Anomalous pulmonary venous drainage**.

Pressure Overload
1. **Tricuspid stenosis** — N.B. in tricuspid atresia a shunt must exist to preserve life. This decompresses the right atrium, so that it is not large (typically a straight right heart border).
2. **Myxoma of the right atrium** — may cause tricuspid obstruction.

Secondary to Right Ventricular Failure
See section 5.4.

5.4   Enlarged Right Ventricle

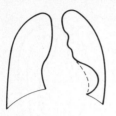

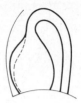

PA
Prominent left heart
border
Elevated apex

Lateral
Prominent anterior part
of cardiac shadow

Secondary to Left Heart Failure/Mitral Valve Disease
See section 5.6.

Pulmonary Arterial Hypertension
1. **Diffuse lung disease** — e.g. chronic obstructive airways disease, interstitial fibrosis, cystic fibrosis, etc.
2. **Pulmonary emboli** — see Pulmonary embolic disease*.
3. **Chronic left to right shunt** — with pulmonary hypertension and right ventricular failure.
4. **Vasculitis** — e.g. polyarteritis nodosa.
5. **Idiopathic** — mostly young females.

Pressure Overload
1. **Pulmonary stenosis**.

Volume Overload
1. **ASD**.
2. **VSD**.

5.5 Enlarged Left Atrium

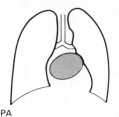

PA
1 Prominent left atrial appendage
2 'Double' right heart border
3 Increased density due to left atrium
4 Splaying of carina and elevated left main bronchus

Lateral
1 Prominent posterosuperior part of cardiac shadow
2 Prominent left atrial impression on oesophagus during barium swallow

Volume Overload
1. **Mitral incompetence**.
2. **VSD**.
3. **PDA**.
4. **ASD with shunt reversal** — Eisenmenger's complex or tricuspid atresia.

Pressure Overload
1. **Mitral stenosis**.
2. **Myxoma of the left atrium**.

Secondary to Left Ventricular Failure

5.6   Enlarged Left Ventricle

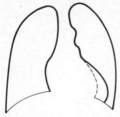 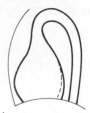

PA
1   Prominent left heart border
2   Rounding of left heart border
3   Apex displaced inferiorly

Lateral
Prominent posteroinferior
part of cardiac shadow

Myocardial
1. **Ischaemia**.
2. **Cardiomyopathy/myocarditis**.

Volume Overload
1. **Aortic incompetence**.
2. **Mitral incompetence**.
3. **VSD**.
4. **PDA**.

High Output States
1. **Anaemia**.
2. **Hyperthyroidism**.
3. **Paget's disease***.
4. **AV fistula**.

Pressure Overload (dilatation is end stage)
1. **Aortic stenosis**.
2. **Hypertension**.
3. **Coarctation of the aorta**.

5.7   Bulge on the Left Heart Border

1. **Enlarged left atrial appendage**.
2. **Ventricular aneurysm**.
3. **Pericardial cyst**.
4. **Pericardial sac defect**.
5. **Myocardial mass** — e.g. neoplasm, hydatid.
6. **Coronary artery aneurysm**.

5.8   Cardiac Calcification

Pericardial
1. **Post-pericarditis** — TB, rheumatic fever, pyogenic, viral.
2. **Post-traumatic/postoperative**.
3. **Uraemia**.
4. **Asbestosis*** } may appear to be 'pericardial'.
5. **Coronary artery**

Myocardial
1. **Calcified infarct**.
2. **Aneurysm**.
3. **Post-myocarditis** — especially rheumatic fever.
4. **Hydatid**.

Intracardiac
1. **Calcified valve** — see section 5.9.
2. **Calcified thrombus** — overlying an infarct or in an aneurysm.
3. **Atrial myxoma** — larger, more mobile and lobulated than a calcified thrombus.

5.9   Valve Calcification

Aortic Valve
1. **Bicuspid aortic valve**.
2. **Rheumatic heart disease**.
3. **Ageing**.
4. **Syphilis**.
5. **Ankylosing spondylitis***.

Mitral Valve
1. **Rheumatic heart disease**.

Pulmonary Valve
1. **Pulmonary valve stenosis** ⎫ in middle age.
2. **Fallot's tetralogy**   ⎭
3. **Pulmonary hypertension**.
4. **Homograft** — for severe Fallot's tetralogy or pulmonary atresia.

Tricuspid Valve
1. **Pulmonary valve stenosis** (with high systolic pressures).
2. **ASD**.
3. **Isolated tricuspid regurgitation**.

5.10 Large Aortic Arch

1. **Unfolded (atherosclerotic) aorta** — parallel walls ± calcification.
2. **Hypertension** — on its own only leads to slight unfolding with left ventricular enlargement.
3. **Aortic incompetence** — prominent ascending aorta.
4. **Aortic stenosis** — post-stenotic dilatation. ± aortic valve calcification.
5. **Aneurysm** — loss of parallelism of walls. Aetiologies include
   (a) Atherosclerosis — calcification prominent.
   (b) Trauma.
   (c) Infection — e.g. syphilis, subacute bacterial endocarditis.
   (d) Intrinsic abnormality — e.g. Marfan's syndrome.
   Macroscopically the aneurysm may be
   (a) Fusiform.
   (b) Saccular.
   (c) Dissecting — signs on the plain chest X-ray include
      (i) Ill-defined aortic outline (because of mediastinal haematoma).
      (ii) Tracheal shift.
      (iii) Left pleural effusion (haemothorax).
      (iv) Left apical cap (also due to effusion).
      (v) Sudden increase in size of the aorta when compared with a previous film.
6. **PDA**.

Further Reading

Dow J., Roebuck E.J. & Cole F. (1970) Dissecting aneurysms of the aorta. *Br. J. Radiol.*, 39: 915–27.

5.11 Small Aortic Arch

1. **Decreased cardiac output** — e.g. mitral stenosis, HOCM.
2. **Intracardiac left to right shunt**.
3. **Coarctation** — long segment 'infantile' type.
4. (**Transposition of great arteries** — rotated but not small.)

5.12   Right-sided Aortic Arch

1. Aortic knuckle on right side.
2. Absent left sided aortic knuckle.
3. Trachea central or slightly to left side.

1. **Fallot's tetralogy** — a feature in 25% of cases.
2. **Pulmonary atresia with a VSD** — 25%.
3. **Transposition of the great vessels** — 20%.
4. **Uncomplicated VSD** — 3%.
5. **Tricuspid atresia** — 5%.
6. **Truncus arteriosus** — 50%.

5.13   Enlarged Superior Vena Cava

Volume Overload
1. **Tricuspid incompetence**.
2. **TAPVD** — if supracardiac. 'Cottage loaf' cardiac configuration, with pulmonary pleonaemia.

Obstruction
1. **Carcinoma of the bronchus**
2. **Mediastinal mass**.
3. **Mediastinal fibrosis** — radiotherapy, idiopathic.
4. **Constrictive pericarditis**.

5.14   Enlarged Azygos Vein

If greater than 1 cm. in diameter. (A normal or abnormal azygos vein will decrease in size in the erect position, on deep inspiration, and during a Valsalva manoeuvre.)

1. **Heart failure**.
2. **Portal hypertension**.
3. **Superior or inferior vena cava obstruction**.
4. **Pregnancy**.
5. **Constrictive pericarditis/pericardial effusion**.

Differential Diagnosis
1. **Sinus venosus defect** — Right upper and middle lobe pulmonary veins drain into the superior vena cava (+ASD).

5.15   Enlarged Pulmonary Arteries

Volume Overload (enlarged central and peripheral vessels)
1. **Left-to-right shunt** — the sign is apparent when the shunt reaches 3:1.
2. **Hyperdynamic circulation** — e.g. thyrotoxicosis, severe anaemia, beri-beri and Paget's disease

Peripheral Arterial Vasoconstriction (enlarged central vessels only)
1. **Hypoxia**—e.g. due to chronic obstructive airways disease or cystic fibrosis.
2. **Secondary to pulmonary venous hypertension** — e.g. mitral stenosis or left ventricular failure.
3. **Secondary to left-to-right shunts**.

Peripheral Arterial Obliteration (enlarged central vessels only)
1. **Secondary to left-to-right shunts**.
2. **Thromboembolic disease** (see Pulmonary embolic disease*).
3. **Tumour emboli**.
4. **Schistosomiasis**.
5. **Vasculitides** — e.g. polyarteritis nodosa.
6. **Idiopathic pulmonary arterial hypertension** — typically in young females.

5.16   Enlarged Pulmonary Veins

Left Ventricular Failure

Obstruction at Mitral or Atrial Level
1. **Mitral stenosis**.
2. **Left atrial myxoma**.
3. **Ball-valve thrombus**.
4. **Cor triatriatum**.

Obstruction Proximal to the Atrium
1. **TAPVD**.
2. **Constrictive pericarditis** — rarely.
3. **Mediastinal fibrosis**.

5.17   Neonatal Pulmonary Venous Congestion

1. Prominent interstitial markings.
2. Indistinct vessels.
3. Perihilar haze.
4. Pleural effusions.
5. Cardiomegaly — in all except the infradiaphragmatic type of TAPVD.

1st Week
1. **Overhydration** — delayed clamping of the cord and twin–twin transfusion.
2. **Asphyxia** — the most common cause of cardiomegaly on the first day.
3. **Hypoplastic left heart**.
4. **Critical aortic stenosis**.
5. **TAPVD (obstructed)**.

2nd–3rd Weeks
1. **Coarctation of the aorta**.
2. **Interrupted aortic arch**.
3. **Critical aortic stenosis**.

4th–6th Weeks
1. **Coarctation**.
2. **Critical aortic stenosis**.
3. **Endocardial fibroelastosis**.
4. **Anomalous left coronary artery**.

N.B. Left-to-right shunts are usually asymptomatic during the neonatal period because of the high pulmonary vascular resistance. However, pulmonary vascular resistance in premature infants is lower, so shunts may present earlier in this particular group. Patent ductus arteriosus is the commonest shunt to cause heart failure in premature infants.

5.18   Neonatal Cyanosis

With Pleonaemia
Cyanosis and congestive cardiac failure — either may predominate.

1. **Transposition**.
2. **Truncus arteriosus**.
3. **TAPVD**.
4. **Single ventricle**.
5. **Hypoplastic left ventricle**
6. **Interrupted aortic arch**

} predominantly congestive cardiac failure, but may be cyanosed.

With Oligaemia and Cardiomegaly
All have an ASD.

1. **Pulmonary stenosis**.
2. **Ebstein's anomaly**.
3. **Pulmonary atresia** with an intact ventricular septum.
4. **Tricuspid atresia**.

With Oligaemia but no Cardiomegaly
Signs sppear towards the end of the first week due to closure of the ductus arteriosus.

1. **Fallot's tetralogy**.
2. **Pulmonary atresia** with a VSD.
3. **Tricuspid atresia**.

See also 'Neonatal respiratory distress', section 4.45.

5.19   Cardiovascular Involvement in Syndromes

Cri-du-chat	Variable.
Down's*	AV canal, VSD, PDA, ASD, and aberrant right subclavian artery.
Ehlers–Danlos	Dissecting aortic aneurysm and intracranial aneurysms.
Ellis–Van Creveld	ASD and common atrium.
Friedreich's ataxia	Hypertrophic cardio-myopathy.
Holt–Oram	ASD and VSD.
Homocystinuria*	Medial degeneration of the aorta and pulmonary artery causing dilatation. Arterial and venous thromboses.
Hurler's/Hunter's*	Intimal thickening of coronary arteries and valves.
Kartagener's	Situs inversus ± septal defects.
Marfan's*	Cystic medial necrosis of the wall of the aorta, and less commonly the pulmonary artery, leading to dilatation and predisposing to dissection. Aortic and mitral regurgitation.
Morquio's*	Late onset of aortic regurgitation.
Noonan's	Pulmonary valve stenosis and septal defects.
Osteogenesis imperfecta*	Aortic and mitral regurgitation. Ruptured chordae.
Rubella	Septal defects, PDA, pulmonary artery branch stenoses and myocardial disease.
Trisomy 13	VSD, ASD, PDA and dextroposition.
Trisomy 18	VSD, ASD and PDA.
Tuberous sclerosis*	Cardiomyopathy and rhabdomyoma of the heart.
Turner's	Coarctation, aortic and pulmonary stenosis.

Bibliography

Felson B. (ed.) (1969) The myocardium. *Semin. Roentgenol.*, 4(4).

Felson B. (ed.) (1979) Acquired valvular disease of the heart. *Semin. Roentgenol.*, 14(2).

Hipona F.A. (ed.) (1971) Cardiac radiology, medical aspects. *Radiol. Clin. North Am.*, 9(3).

Hipona F.A. (ed.) (1971) Cardiac radiology, surgical aspects. *Radiol. Clin. North Am.*, 9(2).

Jefferson K. (1970) The plain chest radiograph in congenital heart disease. *Br. J. Radiol.*, 43: 753–70.

Jefferson K. & Rees S. (1980) *Clinical Cardiac Radiology*, 2nd edn. London: Butterworths.

Möes C.A.F. (1975) Analysis of the chest in the neonate with congenital heart disease. *Radiol. Clin. North Am.*, 13: 251–76.

Sutton D. (ed.) (1980) *Textbook of Radiology and Imaging*, 3rd edn, chaps 22–28. Edinburgh: Churchill Livingstone.

Chapter 6
Abdomen and
Gastrointestinal Tract

6.1 Extraluminal Intra-abdominal Gas

1. **Pneumoperitoneum** (q.v.) — see section 6.2.
2. **Gas in bowel wall**
   (a) Pneumatosis coli.
   (b) Linear pneumatosis intestinalis — infarction (e.g. due to vascular disease, volvulus, necrotizing enterocolitis).
3. **Bilary tree gas** (q.v.) — see section 7.3.
4. **Portal vein gas** (q.v.) — see section 7.4.
5. **Urinary tract gas** (q.v.) — see section 8.4.
6. **Abscess** — mottled gas which may mimic gas within colonic faeces. A homogeneous gas distribution (less common) may mimic gas in normal bowel. Lack of mucosal pattern helps to differentiate it.
7. **Necrotic tumour** — especially following chemotherapy, radiotherapy and therapeutic embolization.
8. **Retroperitoneal gas** — small 'bubbles' or linear translucencies. Secondary to perforation or post-nephrectomy.

Further Reading
Rice R.P., Thompson W.M. & Gedgandas R.K. (1982) The diagnosis and significance of extraluminal gas in the abdomen. *Radiol. Clin. North Am.* 20: 819–37.

6.2   Pneumoperitoneum

1. Erect — Free gas under diaphragm or liver. Can detect 10 ml of air. Can take 10 min for all gas to rise.
2. Supine — Gas outlines both sides of bowel wall, which then appears as a white line. In infants a large volume of gas will collect centrally producing a rounded, relative translucency over the central abdomen. The falciform ligament may also be outlined by free gas. This is seen as a characteristic curvilinear white line in the right upper abdomen.

1. **Perforation**
   (a) Peptic ulcer — 30% do not have free air visible.
   (b) Inflammation — diverticulitis, appendicitis, toxic megacolon, necrotizing enterocolitis.
   (c) Infarction.
   (d) Malignant neoplasms.
   (e) Obstruction.
   (f) Pneumatosis coli — the cysts may rupture.
2. **Iatrogenic (surgery; peritoneal dialysis)** — may take 3 weeks to reabsorb (faster in obese and children), but serial views will show progressive diminution in volume of free air.
3. **Pneumomediastinum** (q.v.) — see section 4.37.
4. **Introduction per vagina** — e.g. douching.
5. **Pneumothorax** — due to a congenital pleuroperitoneal fistula.
6. **Idiopathic**.

6.3   Gasless Abdomen

Adult
1. **High obstruction**.
2. **Ascites** (q.v.) — see section 6.4.
3. **Pancreatitis** (acute) — due to excess vomiting.
4. **Fluid-filled bowel** — closed-loop obstruction, total active colitis, mesenteric infarction (early), bowel wash-out.
5. **Large abdominal mass** — pushes bowel laterally.
6. **Normal**.

Child
1. **High obstruction**
   (a) Duodenal atresia.
   (b) Annular pancreas.
   (c) Volvulus (secondary to malrotation).
   (d) Hypertrophic pyloric stenosis.
   (e) Choledochal cyst.
2. **Vomiting** — including excess naso-gastric aspiration.
3. **Fluid filled bowel** — see above.
4. **Congenital diaphragmatic hernia** — bowel in the chest.

6.4   Ascites

1. Hazy appearance of entire abdomen.
2. Bowel gas 'floats' centrally on supine film.
3. Bulging flank lines.

1. **Cirrhosis**.
2. **Tumours**.
   (a) Malignant — peritoneal metastases, primary carcinoma (particularly ovary and gastrointestinal tract).
   (b) Benign — fibroma of ovary (Meig's syndrome).
3. **Hypoalbuminaemia** — e.g. nephrotic syndrome.
4. **Peritonitis** — particularly TB.
5. **Increased pressure in vascular system distal to liver** — congestive cardiac failure, constrictive pericarditis, thrombosis of inferior vena cava.
6. **Lymphatic obstruction** — chylous ascites, lymphoma, radiation, trauma or filariasis.

6.5   Abdominal Mass in a Neonate

(After Kirks et al., 1981.)

Renal (55%) (q.v.)
1. **Hydronephrosis** (25%) — e.g. posterior urethral valves, ectopic ureterocoele, 'prune-belly', pelviureteric junction obstruction.
2. **Multicystic kidney** (15%).
3. **Infantile polycystic kidneys** (see Polycystic disease*) — ± hepatic fibrosis.
4. **Mesoblastic nephroma** — benign hamartoma.
5. **Renal vein thrombosis** (q.v.) — complication of dehydration/sepsis.
6. **Renal ectopia**.
7. **Wilms' tumour**.

Genital (15%)
1. **Hydrometrocolpos** — dilated fluid-filled vagina and/or uterus, due to vaginal stenosis. Associated with imperforate anus and gastrointestinal fistula.
2. **Ovarian cyst**.

Gastrointestinal (15%) — commonly associated with obstruction.
1. **Duplication** — commonest bowel mass in neonate. Commonly in right lower quadrant.
2. **Mesenteric cyst**.

Non-renal Retroperitoneal (10%)
1. **Adrenal haemorrhage** — relatively common. Due to neonatal stress. ± asymptomatic.
2. **Neuroblastoma**.
3. **Teratoma**.

Hepato/spleno/biliary (5%)
1. **Hepatoblastoma**.
2. **Hepatic cyst**.
3. **Splenic haematoma**.
4. **Choledochal cyst**.

Further Reading
Kirks D.R., Merten D.F., Grossman H. & Bowie J.D. (1981)
    Diagnostic imaging of paediatric abdominal masses: an over-
    view. *Radiol. Clin. North Am.*, 19: 527–45.

See also 'Renal mass in the newborn and young infant', section
8.14.

6.6   Abdominal Mass in a child

(After Kirks et al., 1981.)

Renal (55%)
1. **Wilms' tumour** (22%) — commonest primary abdominal
   neoplasm in childhood (just ahead of neuroblastoma).
   Age: peak incidence at 3 years.
   Site: bilateral in 5%.
   Clinical: usually asymptomatic; most have hyper-
      tension; haematuria in 20%.
   Signs on IVU: 5% calcify; mass causes pelvicalyceal
      distortion; 10% non-functioning.
   Spread: lung commonest (10–15% at presentation); liver
      less common and bone is rare; 5% extend into renal vein
      and inferior vena cava.
   Associated: hemihypertrophy and aniridia.
   Prognosis: good.
2. **Hydronephrosis** (20%) (q.v.).
3. **Cysts** (q.v.).

Non-renal Retroperitoneal (23%)
1. **Neuroblastoma** (21%) —
   Age: usually less than 3 years.
   Site: can occur anywhere in sympathetic chain; 65% in adrenal gland; 5% in pelvis; remainder in thoracic or cervical sympathetic chain.
   Clinical: often present with metastases; symptoms due to local invasion, metastases or catecholamine production.
   Signs on IVU: 50% calcify; mass causes pelvicalyceal displacement; commonly crosses the mid-line.
   Spread: bone, liver, skin, orbit, skull, sutures, nodes.
   Prognosis: poor; in 5% of patients aged less than 1 year, spontaneous cure may occur. A fully differentiated form (ganglioneuroma) may behave as a benign tumour.
2. **Teratoma** (1%) — presacral, 60% calcify. Benign, but malignant change can occur.

Gastrointestinal (18%)
1. **Appendix abscess** (10%) — particularly spreads to pouch anterior to rectum.
2. **Hepatoblastoma** — more commonly in right lobe, but 40% in both lobes. 40% calcify. Arteriography important to define lobar extent.
3. **Haemangioma** — commonly multiple, involving entire liver. Rarely calcify. ± associated with congestive heart failure, and cutaneous haemangiomas.
4. **Choledochal cyst** — the classical triad of mass, pain and jaundice is only present in 10%. Usually affects the supraduodenal portion of common duct. A radioisotope HIDA (hydroxyiminodiacetic acid) scan is diagnostic.

Genital (4%)
1. **Ovarian teratoma** — over 50% calcify. (± teeth/bone).

Further Reading
Kirks D.R., Merten D.F., Grossman H. & Bowie J.D. (1981) Diagnostic imaging of paediatric abdominal masses: an overview. *Radiol. Clin. North Am.*, 19: 527–45.

6.7   Intestinal Obstruction in a Neonate

Duodenal — most common
1. **Stenosis/atresia** — 'double bubble' sign, which may also be seen by ultrasound of fetus (+ hydramnios). Associated with annular pancreas (20%), mongolism (30%) and other abnormalities of gastrointestinal tract (60%).
2. **Annular pancreas** — if not associated with duodenal atresia it may not present until adulthood.
3. **Congenital fibrous band (of Ladd)** — connects caecum to posterolateral abdominal wall and commonly crosses the duodenum. May be complicated by malrotation and mid-gut volvulus.
4. **Congenital web**.
5. **Choledochal cyst**.
6. **Preduodenal portal vein**.

Jejunal
1. **Malrotation and volvulus**.
2. **Atresia** — 50% associated with atretic sites distally (ileum > colon).

Ileal
1. **Meconium ileus** — mottled lucencies due to gas trapped in meconium but only few fluid levels (since it is very viscous). Rapid appearance of fluid levels suggests volvulus. Peritoneal calcification due to perforation occurring in-utero is seen in 30%. Secondary microcolon.
2. **Atresia**.
3. **Inguinal hernia**.
4. **Inspissated milk** — presents 3 days – 6 weeks of age. Dense, amorphous intraluminal masses frequently surrounded by a rim of air, ± mottled lucencies within them. Usually resolves spontaneously.
5. **Paralytic ileus** — e.g. due to drugs administered during labour.

Colonic
1. **Hirschsprung's disease**.
2. **Functional immaturity** — including meconium plug syndrome and small left colon syndrome.
3. **Imperforate anus**
   (a) High — ± sacral agenesis and gas in the bladder (due to a recto-vesical fistula).
   (b) Low — ± perineal fistula.
4. **Atresia**.

Further Reading

Carty H. & Brereton R.J. (1983) The distended neonate. *Clin. Radiol.*, 34: 367–80.
LeQuesne G.W. & Reilly B.J. (1975) Functional immaturity of the large bowel. *Radiol. Clin. North Am.*, 13: 331–42.
Martin D.J. (1975) Experiences with acute surgical conditions. *Radiol. Clin. North Am.*, 13: 297–329.

6.8 Haematemesis

Oesophagus
1. **Hiatus hernia**.
2. **Varices** — 20% of cases are bleeding from a coexisting peptic ulcer.
3. **Neoplasms**.
4. **Mallory–Weiss tears**.

Stomach
1. **Ulcer**.
2. **Erosions** — may be associated with steroids, analgesics or alcohol.
3. **Carcinoma**.

Duodenum
1. **Ulcer**.

Others
1. **Blood dyscrasias**.
2. **Osler–Weber–Rendu (hereditary telangiectasia)** — autosomal dominant. Telangiectasis not prominent until age 20. Epistaxis is often the first symptom.
3. **Connective tissue disorders** — Ehlers–Danlos syndrome, pseudoxanthoma elasticum.

6.9   Dysphagia — Adult

Intrinsic
1. **Reflux stricture**.
2. **Tumours — carcinoma, lymphoma, leiomyoma.**
3. **Ingestion** — corrosive, lye, foreign body.
4. **Iatrogenic** — radiotherapy, prolonged nasogastric intubation.
5. **Plummer–Vinson web** — narrow anterior indentation. Can occur from C4 to T1. Females with iron deficiency anaemia; males post-gastrectomy. Premalignant, but tumour can occur at different site.
6. **Schatzki ring** — marks the squamo-columnar junction lying above the diaphragm. Acute obstruction may occur if internal diameter is less than 6 mm.
7. **Monilia** — painful dysphagia. Can involve entire oesophagus — 'shaggy', ulcerated. Immunosuppression, long-term antibiotics, hypoparathyroidism and debilitation all predispose. Herpes simplex and CMV may cause identical changes.
8. **Skin disorders** — epidermolysis bullosa and pemphigus can produce strictures.

Extrinsic
1. **Tumours** — lymph nodes, mediastinal tumours.
2. **Vascular** — aortic aneurysm; aberrant right subclavian artery (posterior indentation); aberrant left pulmonary artery (anterior indentation); right-sided aortic arch (right lateral and posterior indentation).
3. **Pharyngeal pouch** — ± air/fluid level in neck. Can cause superior mediastinal mass. Signs of aspiration on chest X-ray.
4. **Goitre**.
5. **Enterogenous cyst** — adjacent to, but rarely communicates with, the oesophagus. Hemivertebra and anterior meningocoele may be associated (neuro-enteric cyst).
6. **Prevertebral abscess/haematoma**.

Neuromuscular
1. **Achalasia**.
2. **Scleroderma***.
3. **Chagas' disease**.
4. **Myasthenia gravis**.
5. **Bulbar/pseudobulbar palsy**.

Psychiatric
1. **Globus hystericus**.

6.10   Dysphagia — Neonate

1. **Cleft palate**.
2. **Macroglossia/glossoptosis** — e.g. Beckwith–Wiedemann syndrome and Pierre Robin syndrome.
3. **Oesophageal atresia**.
4. **Vascular rings**.

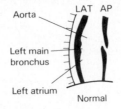

Normal

Aberrant right subclavian artery

Right-sided aortic arch

Aberrant left pulmonary artery

Appearances at barium swallow of the most common vascular rings.

5. **Choanal atresia**.
6. **Neuromuscular defects** — e.g. delayed maturation, prematurity and mental subnormality.

Further Reading

Illingworth R.S. (1969) Sucking and swallowing difficulties in infancy. Diagnostic problems of dysphagia. *Arch. Dis. Child.*, 44: 655–65.

6.11 Oesophageal Strictures — Smooth

Inflammatory

1. **Peptic** — the stricture develops relatively late. Most frequently at the oesophagogastric junction and associated with reflux and a hiatus hernia. Less commonly, more proximal in the oesophagus and associated with heterotopic gastric mucosa (Barrett's oesophagus). ± ulceration.

2. **Scleroderma*** — reflux through a wide open cardia may produce stricture. Oesophagus is the commonest internal organ to be affected. Peristalsis is poor, cardia wide open and the oesophagus dilated (contains air in the resting state).

3. **Corrosives** — acute — oedema, spasm, ulceration and loss of mucosal pattern at 'hold-up' points (aortic arch and oesophago-gastric junction). Strictures are typically long and symmetrical, may take several years to develop and are more likely to be produced by alkalis than acid.

4. **Iatrogenic** — prolonged use of a naso-gastric tube. Stricture in distal oesophagus probably secondary to reflux.

Neoplastic

1. **Carcinoma** — squamous carcinoma may infiltrate submucosally. The absence of a hiatus hernia and the presence of an extrinsic soft-tissue mass should differentiate it from a peptic stricture but a carcinoma arising around the cardia may predispose to reflux.

2. **Mediastinal tumours** — carcinoma of the bronchus and lymph nodes. Localized obstruction ± ulceration and an extrinsic soft-tissue mass.

3. **Leiomyoma** — narrowing due to a smooth, eccentric, polypoid mass. ± central ulceration.

Others

1. **Achalasia** — 'rat-tail' tapering may mimic a stricture; this occurs below the diaphragm. Considerable oesophageal dilatation with food in the lumen.

2. **Skin disorders** — epidermolysis bullosa, pemphigus.

6.12   Oesophageal Strictures — Irregular

Neoplastic

1. **Carcinoma** — increased incidence in achalasia, Plummer–Vinson syndrome, Barrett's oesophagus, coeliac disease, asbestosis, lye ingestion and tylosis. Mostly squamous carcinomas; adenocarcinoma is rare. Appearance include
   (a) Irregular filling defect — annular or eccentric.
   (b) Extraluminal soft tissue mass.
   (c) Re-entrant angles at its margins (shouldering).
   (d) Ulceration.
   (e) Proximal dilatation.
2. **Leiomyosarcoma**.
3. **Carcinosarcoma** — big polypoid tumour ± pedunculated. Better prognosis than squamous carcinoma.
4. **Lymphoma*** — usually extension from gastric involvement.

Inflammatory

1. **Reflux** — rarely irregular.
2. **Crohn's disease*** — rare.

Iatrogenic

1. **Radiotherapy** — rare, unless treating an oesophageal carcinoma. Dysphagia post radiotherapy is usually due to a motility disorder. Acute oesophagitis may occur with a dose of 50–60 Gy (5000–6000 rad).
2. **Fundoplication**.

6.13   Oesophageal Ulceration

Inflammatory
1. **Reflux oesophagitis**.
2. **Barrett's oesophagus**.
3. **Infections** — monilia, herpes or CMV.
4. **Corrosives** (acute).
5. **Radiotherapy** (acute).
6. **Crohn's disease***.

Neoplastic
1. **Carcinoma**.
2. **Leiomyosarcoma and leiomyoma**.
3. **Lymphoma***.
4. **Melanoma**.

6.14   Pharyngeal/Oesophageal 'Diverticula'

Upper Third
1. **Pouch (Zenker's)** — posteriorly, usually on left side, between the fibres of the inferior constrictor and crico-pharyngeus. Can cause dysphagia, regurgitation, aspiration and hoarseness ± an air/fluid level. If large, can appear as a superior mediastinal mass. Food residue within it seen as 'mobile' filling defects.
2. **Lateral pharyngocoele**
    (a) Congenital — remnant of the second branchial arch. Wide mouth (may not retain barium and so may only be seen in recumbent position).
    (b) Acquired — glassblower, trumpeter, etc.

Middle Third
1. **Traction** — at level of carina. May be related to fibrosis after treatment for TB. Asymptomatic.
2. **Developmental** — failure to complete closure of tracheo-oesophageal communication.
3. **Intramural** — very rare. Multiple.

Lower Third
1. **Epiphrenic**.
2. **Ulcer** — peptic or related to steroids, immunosuppression and radiotherapy.
3. **Mucosal tears** — Mallory–Weiss syndrome, post-oesophagoscopy.
4. **Post-Heller's operation**.

Further Reading

Schwartz E.E., Tucker J.A. and Holt G.P. (1981) Cervical dysphagia: pharyngeal protrusions and achalasia. *Clin. Radiol.*, 32: 643–50.

6.15   Tertiary Contractions in the Oesophagus

Unco-ordinated, non-propulsive contractions.

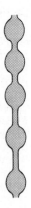

1. **Reflux oesophagitis**.
2. **Presbyoesophagus** — impaired motor function due to muscle atrophy in the elderly. Occurs in 25% of people over 60 years.
3. **Obstruction at the cardia** — from any cause.
4. **Neuropathy**
    (a) Early achalasia — before dilatation occurs.
    (b) Diabetes.
    (c) Alcoholism.
    (d) Malignant infiltration.
    (e) Chagas' disease.

6.16   Stomach Masses and Filling Defects

Primary Malignant Neoplasms

1. **Carcinoma** — most polypoidal carcinomas are 1–4 cm in diameter. (Any polyp greater than 2 cm in diameter must be considered to be malignant.) Granular/lobulated surface pattern is suggestive of carcinoma. Asbestosis, adenomatous polyps and Peutz–Jeghers' syndrome predispose. Metastases may calcify and sclerotic or lytic bone metastases may occur.

2. **Lymphoma*** — primary gastric lymphoma is usually non-Hodgkin's. It can be ulcerative and infiltrative as well as polypoid. Often cannot distinguish it from carcinoma, but extension across the pylorus is suggestive of a lymphoma.

Polyps

1. **Hyperplastic** — accounts for most polyps. Usually multiple, small (less than 1 cm in diameter) and occur randomly throughout stomach but predominantly affect body and fundus. Associated with chronic gastritis.

2. **Adenomatous** — usually solitary, 1–4 cm in diameter, sessile and occur in antrum. High incidence of malignant transformation (particularly if greater than 2 cm in size) and carcinomas elsewhere in stomach (because of dysplastic epithelium). Associated with pernicious anaemia.

3. **Hamartomatous** — characteristically multiple, small and relatively spare the antrum. Occur in 30% of Peutz–Jeghers' syndrome, 40% of familial polyposis coli and Gardner's syndrome.

Submucosal Neoplasms

Smooth, well-defined filling defect, with a re-entry angle.

1. **Leiomyoma** — commonest by far. Can be very large with a substantial exogastric component. Central ulceration and massive haematemesis may occur.

2. **Lipoma** — can change shape with position of patient and may be relatively mobile on palpation.

3. **Neurofibroma** — N.B. Leiomyomas and lipomas are more common, even in patients with generalized neurofibromatosis.

4. **Metastases** — Frequently ulcerate — 'bulls eye' lesion (q.v.). Usually melanoma, but bronchus, breast, lymphoma, Kaposi's sarcoma and any adenocarcinoma may metastasize to stomach. Breast primary often produces a scirrhous reaction in the distal part of the stomach which is indistinguishable from linitis plastica (q.v.).

Extrinsic Indentation
1. **Pancreatic tumour/pseudocyst**.
2. **Splenomegaly/hepatomegaly**.
3. **Retroperitoneal tumours**.

Others
1. **Nissen fundoplication** — may mimic a distorted mass in the fundus.
2. **Bezoar** — 'mass' is mobile. Tricho- (hair) or phyto- (vegetable matter).
3. **Pancreatic rest** — ectopic pancreatic tissue causes a small filling defect, usually on the inferior wall of the antrum, and resembles a submucosal tumour. Central 'blob' of barium ('bull's eye' or target lesion) in 50%.

6.17   Thick Stomach Folds

Thickness greater than 1 cm.

Inflammatory

1. **Gastritis** — associated with peptic ulceration.
2. **Zollinger–Ellison syndrome** — suspect if post-bulbar ulcers. Ulceration in both 1st and 2nd parts of duodenum is suggestive, but ulceration distal to this is virtually diagnostic. Thick folds and small bowel dilatation may occur in response to excess acidity.
   Due to gastrinoma of non-beta cells of pancreas (no calcification, moderately vascular). 50% malignant — metastases to liver. (10% of gastrinomas may be ectopic — usually in medial wall of the duodenum.)
3. **Pancreatitis (acute)**.
4. **Crohn's disease*** — mild thickening of folds with aphthous ulceration may occur in up to 40% of Crohn's. However, these signs are subtle, and more obvious disease (i.e. deformity and narrowing of the antrum) only occurs in 2% of these.

Infiltrative/Neoplastic

1. **Lymphoma*** — usually non-Hodgkin's, and may be primary or secondary. Folds, irregular and extend into duodenum in 20% of cases. Stomach remains relatively distensible (c.f. carcinomatous infiltration). Rapid change in size is possible. Ulcerating and polypoid forms may occur.
2. **Carcinoma** — irregular folds with rigid wall.
3. **Pseudolymphoma** — benign reactive lymphoid hyperplasia. 70% have an ulcer near the centre of the area affected.
4. **Eosinophilic gastroenteritis**.

Others

1. **Ménétrier's disease** — smooth folds predominantly on greater curve. Rarely extend into antrum. No rigidity or ulcers. 'Weep' protein sufficient to cause hypoproteinaemia (effusions, oedema, thick folds in small bowel). Commonly achlorhydric — c.f. Zollinger–Ellison syndrome.
2. **Varices** — occur in fundus and usually associated with oesophageal varices.

6.18   Linitis Plastica

Neoplastic
1. **Gastric carcinoma**.
2. **Lymphoma***.
3. **Metastases** — particularly breast.
4. **Local invasion** — pancreatic carcinoma.

Inflammatory
1. **Corrosives** — can cause rigid stricture of antrum extending up to the pylorus.
2. **Radiotherapy** — can cause rigid stricture of antrum with some deformity. Mucosal folds may be thickened or effaced. Large antral ulcers can also occur.
3. **Granulomata** — Crohn's disease, TB.
4. **Eosinophilic enteritis** — commonly involves gastric antrum (causing narrowing and nodules) in addition to small bowel. Blood eosinophilia. Occasionally spares the mucosa, so needs full thickness biopsy for confirmation.

6.19   Gastrocolic Fistula

Inflammatory
1. **Peptic ulcer**.
2. **Crohn's disease***.
3. **Pancreatitis (chronic)**.
4. **Infections** — tuberculosis, actinomycosis.

Neoplastic
1. **Carcinoma** — of stomach, colon or pancreas.
2. **Metastases**.

6.20 Gastric Dilatation

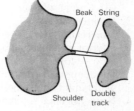

Gas- or food-filled stomach. Mottled translucencies (due to gas trapped in food residue) may be seen in gastric dilatation secondary to chronic obstruction. Resembles heavy faecal loading of the colon.

Mechanical Obstruction
1. **Fibrosis secondary to ulceration** — long history of dyspepsia.
2. **Malignancy** — shorter history, therefore dilatation is usually less marked. Often no abdominal pain.
3. **Volvulus** — 'organo-axial', associated with hiatus hernia. 'Vertical axis', not associated with hiatus hernia.
4. **Infantile hypertrophic pyloric stenosis** — the radiological signs on a barium meal are
   (a) 'String sign' — barium in the narrowed pyloric canal.
   (b) 'Shoulder sign', the pyloric 'tumour' indenting the barium-filled antrum.
   (c) 'Beak sign' — incomplete extension of the barium into the narrowed pyloric channel.
   (d) 'Double track sign' — parallel mucosal folds in the pyloric channel.
5. **Proximal small bowel obstruction** — gastric and small bowel dilatation.

Paralytic Ileus
1. **Postoperative**.
2. **Post-vagotomy**.
3. **Drugs** — e.g. anticholinergics.
4. **Metabolic** — uraemia, hypokalaemia, etc.

Further Reading
Kreel L. & Ellis H. (1965) Pyloric stenosis in adults: a clinical and radiological study of 100 consecutive patients. *Gut*, 6: 253–61.

6.21   'Bull's Eye' (Target) Lesion in the Stomach

Ulcer on apex of a nodule.

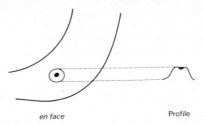

en face   Profile

1. **Submucosal metastases** — may be multiple
   (a) Melanoma — commonest.
   (b) Lymphoma*.
   (c) Carcinoma — breast, bronchus, pancreas.
   (d) Carcinoid.
2. **Leiomyoma**.
3. **Pancreatic 'rest'** — ectopic pancreatic tissue. Usually on inferior wall of antrum. A central 'blob' of barium is seen in 50% — collects in primitive duct remnant. Can also occur in duodenum, jejunum, Meckel's diverticulum, liver, gallbladder and spleen.
4. **Neurofibroma** — may be multiple. Other stigmata of neurofibromatosis.

6.22   Gas in the Stomach Wall

1. **Iatrogenic** — gastroscopy/overdistension.
2. **Pneumatosis cystoides**.
3. **Ischaemia**.
4. **Peptic ulcer with intramural erosion**.
5. **Necrotizing enterocolitis** — neonates. More common in colonic wall — bowel distension, gas in portal venous system (20%). ± perforation with ascites. 25% develop strictures later.

6.23   Cobblestone Duodenal Cap

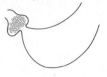

Big 'Polypoid'
1. **Oedema** — associated with an ulcer.
2. **Hypertrophied Brunner's glands** — can extend from pylorus to ampulla of Vater. Uniform in size.
3. **Crohn's disease*** — involved in 2% and may rarely present here. Usually signs present in gastric antrum also.
4. **Varices** — base of cap. Decrease in size in erect position. Invariably associated with oesophageal varices.
5. **Lymphoma***.
6. **Carcinoma**.

Small
1. **Duodenitis** — ± central flecks of barium.
2. **Nodular lymphoid hyperplasia** — pinpoint (1–3 mm) nodules involving the entire duodenal loop. (Duodenum > jejunum.)
3. **Food residue/effervescent granules** — move around.
4. **Heterotopic gastric mucosa** — base of cap, adjacent to pylorus.

Further Reading
Schulman A. (1970) The cobblestone appearance of the duodenal cap, duodenitis and hyperplasia of Brunner's glands. *Br. J. Radiol.*, 43: 787–95.

6.24   Decreased/absent Duodenal Folds

1. **Scleroderma***.
2. **Crohn's disease***.
3. **Strongyloides**.
4. **Cystic fibrosis***.
5. **Amyloidosis**.

6.25   Thickened Duodenal Folds

Inflammatory
1. **Duodenitis**
2. **Pancreatitis**
3. **Crohn's disease*** — occurs before aphthous ulcers. Mild signs occur in duodenum in up to 40%, but severe involvement only occurs in 2%. Cap and proximal half of second part of duodenum predominantly affected.
4. **Zollinger–Ellison syndrome** — response to excess acidity.

Neoplastic
1. **Lymphoma***.
2. **Metastases** — particularly melanoma, breast, ovary, gastrointestinal tract (lung, kidney are rare).

Infiltrative
1. **Amyloidosis** — bowel commonly involved (primary generalized thickening; secondary — segmental thickening).
2. **Eosinophilic enteritis** — gastric antrum commonly involved. Blood eosinophilia.
3. **Mastocytosis** — dense bones. ± gastric polyps.
4. **Whipple's disease**.

Vascular
1. **Intramural haematoma** — due to trauma. Common in the duodenum because it is fixed to the posterior abdominal wall. 'Stacked coins' appearance. An extensive haematoma may occur in bleeding diatheses.
2. **Ischaemia** — widespread changes can occur in vasculitis secondary to radiotherapy, collagen diseases and Henoch–Schönlein purpura.

Oedema
1. **Hypoproteinaemia** — nephrotic syndrome, cirrhosis or protein-losing enteropathy.
2. **Venous obstruction** — cirrhosis, Budd–Chiari syndrome or constrictive pericarditis.
3. **Lymphatic obstruction**.
4. **Angioneurotic oedema**.

Infestations
1. **Worms**
   (a) Hookworm (*Ankylostoma duodenale*) — the head of
       the worm produces an inflammatory reaction.
   (b) Tapeworm (*Taenia saginata* or *T. solium*) — has a
       similar effect on the duodenum. The worm may be
       visible as a filling defect during a barium study.
   (c) Strongyloides — similar appearance to giardiasis (see
       below). Strictures in chronic cases.
2. **Giardiasis** — predominantly affects the duodenum and
   proximal jejunum. Thickened, blunted and distorted
   mucosal folds. Hypermotility leads to rapid transit. Spasm
   produces narrowing. May be associated with nodular
   lymphoid hyperplasia or hypogammaglobulinaemia.

See also sections 6.29 and 6.30.

6.26   Dilated Duodenum

Mechanical Obstruction
1. **Bands** — most frequent cause of neonatal duodenal
   obstruction. Associated with malrotation and midgut
   volvulus.
2. **Atresia, webs, stenosis** — often associated with Down's
   syndrome. 'Double bubble' sign in neonate due to dilated
   stomach and duodenum. Webs have a high incidence of
   incomplete rotation.
3. **Annular pancreas**.
4. **Superior mesenteric artery syndrome** — hold up of barium
   in third part of duodenum with some proximal dilatation
   and vigorous peristalsis (prior to muscle relaxant). Post-
   prandial pain relieved by lying on left side. Associated with
   a plaster of Paris body cast. 20% have associated duodenal
   ulcer. Never occurs in obese people.

Paralytic Ileus — particularly due to pancreatitis.

*Scleroderma**

Further Reading
Anderson J.R., Earnshaw P.M. & Fraser G.M. (1982) Extrinsic
    compression of the third part of the duodenum. *Clin. Radiol.*,
    33: 75–81.

6.27   Dilated Small Bowel

Calibre: proximal jejunum   >   3.5 cm   (4.5 cm if small bowel
enema)
mid-small bowel   >   3.0 cm   (4.0 cm if small bowel
enema)
ileum   >   2.5 cm   (3.0 cm if small bowel enema).

Normal Folds

1. **Mechanical obstruction** —   ± dilated large bowel, depending on level of obstruction.
2. **Paralytic ileus** — dilated small and large bowel.
3. **Coeliac disease, tropical sprue, dermatitis herpetiformis** — can produce identical signs. Dilatation is the hallmark, and correlates well with severity, but it is relatively uncommon. ± dilution and flocculation of barium. See section 6.32.
4. **Scleroderma***.
5. **Iatrogenic** — post-vagotomy and gastrectomy may produce dilatation due to rapid emptying of stomach contents. Dilatation may also occur proximal to a small bowel loop.

Thick Folds

1. **Ischaemia**.
2. **Crohn's disease*** — combination of obstructive and inflammatory changes.
3. **Radiotherapy**.
4. **Lymphoma***.
5. **Zollinger–Ellison syndrome** — ileus due to excess acidity.
6. **Extensive small bowel resection** — compensatory dilatation and thickening of folds.
7. **Amyloidosis**.

6.28   Strictures in the Small Bowel

1. **Adhesions** — angulation of bowel which is constant in site. Normal mucosal folds.
2. **Crohn's disease*** — ± ulcers and altered mucosal pattern.
3. **Ischaemia** — ulcers are rare. Evolution is more rapid than Crohn's ± long strictures.
4. **Radiotherapy** — ulcers are rare, smooth tapering strictures are secondary to vasculitis.
5. **Tumours**
   (a) Lymphoma — usually secondary to contiguous spread from lymph nodes. Primary disease may occur and is nearly always due to non-Hodgkin's lymphoma.
   (b) Carcinoid — although the appendix is the commonest site, these never metastasize. Of those occurring in small bowel, 90% are in ileum (mostly distal 2 feet), and 30% are multifocal. A fibroblastic response to infiltration produces a stricture, ± mass. It is the commonest primary malignancy of small bowel, but only 30% metastasize (more likely if > 2 cm diam.) or invade. Carcinoid syndrome only develops with liver metastases.
   (c) Carcinoma — usually stenosing, rarely polypoidal. More common in jejunum (unless associated with Crohn's disease).
   (d) Sarcoma — lympho- or leiomyo-. Thick folds with eccentric lumen.
   (e) Metastases.
6. **Enteric coated potassium tablets**.

6.29   Thickened Folds in Non-dilated Small Bowel — Smooth and Regular

Fold thickness: jejunum   >   2.5 mm
                   ileum   >   2.0 mm.

Vascular
1. **Intramural haematoma**
    (a) Trauma — commonest in duodenum, since fixed to posterior abdominal wall ('stacked coin' appearance).
    (b) Bleeding diathesis — commonly localized to a few loops.
2. **Ischaemia**
    (a) Acute — embolus, Henoch-Schönlein purpura. Can produce ileus. May perforate. Ulcers rare.
    (b) Chronic — vasculitis (collagen, radiotherapy), atheroma, fibromuscular dysplasia. Present with postprandial pain, and malabsorption.

Radiotherapy
Dose > 50 Gy (5000 rad). Most changes due to vasculitis. Poor correlation of signs with severity of symptoms. Treatment of cervical carcinoma accounts for majority of cases — distal small bowel and distal colon most commonly involved. Most changes are evident in 6 months – 2 years (occasionally takes 10 years).

1. **Acute** — thick folds with rigidity and poor peristalsis on screening. Angulation due to adhesions. ± fistula and obstruction. Ulcers rare (distinguishes it from Crohn's disease). These changes often overlap with chronic fibrotic changes.
2. **Chronic** — strictures due to fibrosis.

Oedema
1. **Adjacent inflammation** — focal.
2. **Hypoproteinaemia** — e.g. nephrotic, cirrhosis, protein losing enteropathy. Generalized.
3. **Venous obstruction** — e.g. cirrhosis, Budd-Chiari syndrome, constrictive pericarditis.
4. **Lymphatic obstruction** — e.g. lymphoma, retroperitoneal fibrosis, primary lymphangiectasia (child with leg oedema).
5. **Angioneurotic**.

Early Infiltration
1. **Amyloidosis** — gastrointestinal tract commonly involved. Primary amyloid tends to produce generalized thickening, whereas secondary amyloid produces focal lesions. Malabsorption is unusual.
2. **Eosinophilic enteritis** — focal or generalized. Gastric antrum frequently involved. No ulcers. Blood eosinophilia. Occasionally spares mucosa — therefore need full thickness biopsy for diagnosis.

Coeliac Disease
Thickening of folds is not common, and is probably a functional abnormality rather than true fold thickening. ± jejunal dilatation.

Abetalipoproteinaemia
Rare, inherited. Malabsorption, acanthocytosis, and CNS abnormality. ± dilated bowel.

6.30 Thickened Folds in Non-dilated Small Bowel — Irregular and Distorted

Fold thickness: jejunum > 2.5 mm
                   ileum   > 2.0 mm

Localized

Inflammatory
1. **Crohn's disease*** — occurs before aphthous ulcers.
2. **Zollinger–Ellison syndrome** — predominantly proximal small bowel. Dilatation may occur.

Neoplastic
1. **Lymphoma***.
2. **Metastases** — particularly melanoma, breast, ovary and gastrointestinal tract.
3. **Carcinoid** — commonest primary malignant small bowel tumour. 90% in the ileum and mostly in the distal 60 cm. It is more common in the appendix, where it is a benign tumour.

Infective
1. **Tuberculosis** — can look identical to Crohn's disease, but predominant caecal involvement may help to distinguish it. Less than 50% have pulmonary tuberculosis.

Widespread

Infiltrative
1. **Amyloidosis**.
2. **Eosinophilic enteritis**.
3. **Mastocytosis** — may have superimposed small nodules, urticaria pigmentosa and sclerotic bone lesions.
4. **Whipple's disease** — flitting arthralgia, lymphadenopathy and sacro-iliitis.

Inflammatory
1. **Crohn's disease***.

Infestations
1. **Giardiasis** — associated with hypogammaglobulinaemia and nodular lymphoid hyperplasia.
2. **Strongyloides** — ± absent folds in chronic cases.

Stomach Abnormality with Thickened Small Bowel Mucosal Folds
1. **Lymphoma/metastases.**
2. **Zollinger–Ellison syndrome.**
3. **Ménétrier's disease.**
4. **Amyloidosis.**
5. **Eosinophilic enteritis.**

Further Reading
Goldberg H.I. & Sheft D.J. (1976) Abnormalities in small intestine contour and calibre. *Radiol. Clin. North Am.*, 14: 461–75.

6.31 Multiple Nodules in the Small Bowel

Inflammatory
1. **Nodular lymphoid hyperplasia** — nodules 2–4 mm with normal fold thickness. Associated with hypogammaglobulinaemia (IgA and IgM). Produces malabsorption, and there is a high incidence of intestinal infections (particularly giardiasis, but strongyloides and monilia may also occur). Can also affect the colon, where in children it may be a normal variant, but in adults it may be an early sign of Crohn's disease.
2. **Crohn's disease*** — 'cobblestone' mucosa but other characteristic signs present.

Infiltrative
1. **Whipple's disease** — ± myriad of tiny (< 1 mm) nodules superimposed on thick folds.
2. **Waldenström's macroglobulinaemia** — ± myriad of tiny (< 1 mm) nodules. Folds usually normal, but may occasionally be thick.
3. **Mastocytosis** — nodules a little larger and folds usually thick.

Neoplastic
1. **Lymphoma*** — can produce diffuse nodules (2–4 mm) of varying sizes. Ulceration in the nodules is not uncommon.
2. **Polyposis**
   (a) Peutz–Jeghers' syndrome — autosomal dominant. Buccal pigmentation. Multiple hamartomas (± intussuscept) 'carpeting' the small bowel. Can also involve the colon (30%) and stomach (25%). Not in themselves premalignant, but associated with carcinoma of stomach, duodenum and ovary.
   (b) Gardner's syndrome — predominantly in the colon. Occasionally has adenomas in small bowel.
   (c) Canada–Cronkhite syndrome — predominantly stomach and colon, but may affect the small bowel.
3. **Metastases** — on antimesenteric border. Particularly melanoma, breast, gastrointestinal tract and ovary. (Rarely bronchus and kidney.) ± ascites.

Infective
1. **Typhoid** — hypertrophy of 'Peyer's patches'.
2. **Yersinia** — ± nodules in terminal ileum.

Further Reading
Marshak R.H., Lindner A.E., & Maklansky D. (1976) Immunoglobulin disorders of the small bowel. *Radiol. Clin. North Am.*, 14: 477–91.

6.32 Malabsorption

Mucosal

1. **Coeliac disease** — commonest cause of malabsorption. Not all have steatorrhea — can present with iron or folate deficiency. Jejunal biopsy shows subtotal villous atrophy (this can also occur in Whipple's disease, primary lymphoma and chronic ulcerative enteritis). Jejunal dilatation is the hallmark, but is relatively uncommon. It correlates well with severity. Fold thickness is normal in uncomplicated coeliac disease. Other signs, which are occasionally demonstrable on a barium follow through examination are
   (a) Dilution of barium, because of hypersecretion of fluid by the bowel.
   (b) Segmentation of the column of barium. This is most marked in the ileum.
   (c) Moulage sign. The appearance of barium in a feature-less tube due to the complete effacement of mucosal folds.
   If bowel calibre increases while on a gluten free diet suspect a complication, i.e. lymphoma, carcinoma or intussusception (rare and non-obstructive). Tropical sprue and dermatitis herpetiformis can present with identical appearances.
2. **Inflammation**
   (a) Crohn's disease*.
   (b) Radiotherapy — if there is widespread involvement.
   (c) Scleroderma* — due to hypomotility.
3. **Ischaemia** — can cause mild malabsorption if chronic and widespread.
4. **Infiltration**
   (a) Whipple's disease.
   (b) Mastocytosis.
   (c) Amyloidosis — particularly in primary amyloidosis, since generalized bowel involvement is more common.
   (d) Eosinophilic enteritis — blood eosinophilia is common.

5. **Lymphangiectasia** — child. Blocked lymphatics interfere with the transport of fat. Hypoproteinaemia due to protein loss into the gut is common.
6. **Parasites** — particularly *Giardia* and *Strongyloides* spp.

Digestive
1. **Gastrectomy**.
2. **Biliary obstruction**.
3. **Pancreatic dysfunction** — pancreatitis, cystic fibrosis, carcinoma and pancreatectomy.
4. **Disaccharidase deficiency** — lactase deficiency is the commonest.

Anatomical
1. **Fistula** — even a small one to the colon allows bacterial colonization.
2. **Resection**.
3. **Stagnant loop/stricture.**
4. **Jejunal diverticulosis** — in the erect view may resemble obstruction with multiple fluid levels. However, the diverticula have smooth walls, i.e. no mucosal folds. Produces folate deficiency.

Further Reading
Laws J.W. & Pitman R.G. (1960) The radiological investigation of the malabsorption syndromes. *Br. J. Radiol.*, 33: 211–22.

6.33 Protein-losing Enteropathy

Oedema in small bowel will occur if plasma albumin $< 20 \ gl^{-1}$.

'Mucosal'
1. **Coeliac disease.**
2. **Ménétrier's disease.**
3. **Sprue.**

Inflammatory
1. **Crohn's disease*.**
2. **Ulcerative colitis*.**
3. **Radiotherapy.**

Ulceration
1. **Carcinoma stomach/colon.**
2. **Villous adenoma.**

Venous Obstruction
1. **Cirrhosis.**
2. **Inferior vena cava thrombosis.**
3. **Constrictive pericarditis.**

Chronic Arterial Obstruction

Lymphatic Obstruction
1. **Lymphangiectasia.**
2. **Lymphoma*.**
3. **Retroperitoneal fibrosis** (q.v.).

Infiltrative
1. **Whipple's disease.**
2. **Eosinophilic enteritis.**

Further Reading
Marshak R.H., Wolf B.S., Cohen N. & Janowitz H.D. (1961) Protein-losing disorders of the gastrointestinal tract: Roentgen features. *Radiology*, 77: 893–905.

6.34   Lesions in the Terminal Ileum

Inflammatory
1. **Crohn's disease***.
2. **Ulcerative colitis*** — 10% of those with total colitis have 'backwash' ileitis for up to 25 cm causing granular mucosa, ± dilatation. No ulcers.
3. **Radiotherapy** — ± strictures and thickened folds. Ulcers rare.

Infective
1. **Tuberculosis** — can look identical to Crohn's disease. Continuity of involvement with caecum and ascending colon can occur. Longitudinal ulcers are uncommon. Less than 50% have pulmonary TB. Caecum is predominantly involved — progressive contraction of caecal wall opposite the ileocaecal valve, and cephalad retraction of the caecum with straightening of the ileocaecal angle.
2. **Yersinia** — 'cobblestone' appearance and aphthous ulcers. No deep ulcers and spontaneous resolution, usually within 10 weeks, distinguishes it from Crohn's disease.
3. **Actinomycosis** — very rare. Predominantly caecum. ± associated bone destruction with periosteal reaction.
4. **Histoplasmosis** — very rare.

Neoplastic
1. **Lymphoma*** — may look like Crohn's disease. (See section 6.28.)
2. **Carcinoid** — appendix is the commonest site. Of those found in the small bowel, the terminal ileum is the commonest site. ± fibrotic stricture and nodules. 30% multifocal. (See section 6.28.)
3. **Metastases** — no ulcers.

Ischaemia
Rare site. Thickened folds, 'cobblestone' appearance and 'thumb printing', but rapid progression of changes helps to discriminate it from Crohn's disease.

Further Reading
Calenoff, L. (1970) Rare ileocaecal lesions. *Am. J. Roentgenol.*, 110: 343–51.

6.35   Colonic Polyps

Adenomatous
1. **Simple tubular adenoma — tubulovillous adenoma — villous adenoma** — these three form a spectrum both in size and degree of dysplasia. Villous adenoma is the largest, shows the most severe dysplasia and has the highest incidence of malignancy. Signs suggestive of malignancy are
   - (a) Size —   < 5 mm   —   0% malignant
     5 mm – 1 cm —   1% malignant
     1–2 cm   — 10% malignant
     > 2 cm   — 50% malignant.
   - (b) Sessile — base greater than height.
   - (c) 'Puckering' of colonic wall at base of polyp.
   - (d) Irregular surface.

   Villous adenomas are typically fronded, sessile and are poorly coated by barium because of their mucous secretion. May cause a protein-losing enteropathy or hypokalaemia.
2. **Familial polyposis coli** — autosomal dominant. Starts in adolescence. Carpets the entire colon with adenomas. Always affects rectum and polyps are more numerous in distal colon. Carcinoma of colon develops in early adulthood. (Has occurred in 30% by 10 years after diagnosis made, and in 100% by 20 years.) 60% of those who present with colonic symptoms already have a carcinoma. The carcinoma is multifocal in 50%. Extra-colonic abnormalities may occur — hamartomas of stomach (40%) and adenomas of duodenum (25%).
3. **Gardner's syndrome** — autosomal dominant. Adenomas of colon (and occasionally small bowel), osteomas of skull and mandible, multiple skin tumours and epidermoid cysts. Same risk of colonic carcinoma as familial polyposis coli. Also, 12% develop carcinoma of duodenum (periampullary). Other tumours associated are carcinomas of thyroid and adrenal, carcinoid, and hamartomas of the stomach. About 5% may develop desmoid tumours of the mesentery or anterior abdominal wall.

Hyperplastic
1. **Solitary/multiple** — most frequently found in rectum.
2. **Nodular lymphoid hyperplasia** — usually children. Filling defects are smaller than familial polyposis coli.

Hamartomatous
1. **Juvenile polyposis** — ± familial. Children under 10. Commonly solitary in rectum.
2. **Peutz–Jeghers' syndrome** — autosomal dominant. 'Carpets' small bowel, but also affects colon and stomach in 30%. Increased incidence of carcinoma of stomach, duodenum and ovary.

Inflammatory
1. **Ulcerative colitis*** — polyps can be seen at all stages of activity of the colitis (no malignant potential): acute — pseudo-polyps (i.e. mucosal hyperplasia); chronic — sessile polyp (resembles villous adenoma); quiescent —tubular/ filiform ('wormlike') and can show a branching pattern.
2. **Crohn's disease*** — polyps less common than in ulcerative colitis.

Infective
1. **Schistosomiasis** — predominantly involves rectum. ± strictures.
2. **Amoebiasis**.

Others
1. **Canada–Cronkhite syndrome** — not hereditary. Predominantly affects stomach and colon, but can occur anywhere in bowel. Increased incidence of carcinoma of colon. Other features are alopecia, nail atrophy and skin pigmentation.
2. **Turcot's syndrome** — autosomal recessive. Increased incidence of CNS malignancy.

Further Reading

Bresnihan E.R. & Simpkins K.C. (1975) Villous adenoma of the large bowel: Benign and malignant. *Br. J. Radiol.*, 48: 801–6.
Dodds W.J. (1976) Clinical and roentgen features of the intestinal polyposis syndromes. *Gastrointest. Radiol.*, 1: 127–42.
Dolan K.D., Seibert J. & Siebart R.W. (1973) Gardner's syndrome. *Am. J. Roentgenol.*, 119: 359–64.
Morson B.C. (1974) The polyp cancer sequence in the large bowel. *Proc. Roy. Soc. Med.*, 67: 451–7.

6.36   Colonic Strictures

Neoplastic
1. **Carcinoma** — mucosal destruction and 'shouldering'. Often shorter than 6 cm.
2. **Lymphoma***.

Inflammatory
Tend to be symmetrical, smooth and tapered.
1. **Ulcerative colitis*** — usually requires extensive involvement for longer than 5 years. Commonest in sigmoid colon. May be multiple. Beware malignant complications — these are commonly irregular, annular strictures (30% are multiple). Risk factors are: total colitis, length of history (risk starts at 10 years and increases by 10% per decade), epithelial dysplasia on biopsy.
2. **Crohn's disease*** — strictures occur in 25% of colonic Crohn's disease, and 50% of these are multiple.
3. **Pericolic abscess** — can look malignant, but relative lack of mucosal destruction.
4. **Radiotherapy** — occurs several years after treatment. Commonest site is rectosigmoid colon, which appears smooth and narrow and rises vertically out of pelvis due to thickening of surrounding tissue.

Ischaemia
Infarction heals by stricture formation relatively rapidly. Commonest site is splenic flexure, but 20% occur in other sites. It can be extensive and has tapering ends.

Infective
1. **Tuberculosis** — commonest in ileocaecal region. Short, 'hourglass' stricture.
2. **Amoeboma** — more common in descending colon. Occurs in 2–8% of amoebiasis and is multiple in 50%. Rapid improvement after treatment with metronidazole.
3. **Schistosomiasis** — commonly rectosigmoid region. Granulation tissue forming after the acute stage (oedema, fold-thickening and polyps) may cause a stricture.

4. **Lymphogranuloma venereum** — sexually transmitted chlamydia. Late complications are strictures which are characteristically long and tubular and affect the recto-sigmoid region. Fistulate may occur.

Extrinsic masses — inflammatory, tumours (primary and secondary), and endometriosis.

Cathartic colon — pseudostrictures which alter their configuration during the barium enema. The colon may be atonic and dilated. Changes are initially in the ascending colon, but can progress to involve all of the colon.

Further Reading

Simpkins K.C. and Young A.C. (1971). The differential diagnoses of large bowel strictures. *Clin. Radiol.*, 22: 449–57.

6.37   Gas in the Wall of the Colon

1. **Toxic megacolon** (q.v.).
2. **Pneumatosis coli** — can produce 'polypoid' filling defects in barium enema which may be large enough to cause obstruction. Some are associated with chronic obstructive airways disease.
3. **Infarction**.
4. **Necrotizing enterocolitis** (neonate).

6.38   Megacolon in an Adult

Colonic calibre greater than 5.5 cm.

Non-toxic (without mucosal abnormalities)
1. **Distal obstruction** — e.g. carcinoma.
2. **Paralytic ileus**.
3. **Electrolyte imbalance**.
4. **Purgative abuse**.

Toxic (with severe mucosal abnormalities)
Deep ulceration and inflammation produce a neuromuscular degeneration. Thick oedematous folds and extensive slough-ing of the mucosa leaves mucosal islands. The underlying causes produce similar plain film changes. The presence of intramural gas indicates that perforation is imminent.
1. **Inflammatory**
   (a) Ulcerative colitis*.
   (b) Crohn's disease*.
   (c) Pseudomembranous colitis.
2. **Ischaemic colitis**.
3. **Dysentery**
   (a) Amoebiasis.
   (b) Salmonella.

6.39   Megacolon in a Child

1. **Hirschsprung's disease** — chronic constipation leads to secondary megacolon.
2. **Functional/psychogenic** — the rectum is distended with faeces.
3. **Cretinism***.
4. **Mechanical obstruction**
   (a) Stricture — e.g. post necrotizing enterocolitis (25%).
   (b) Tumour — e.g. sacrococcygeal teratoma.
   (c) Imperforate anus — in a neonate.
5. **Paralytic ileus** — generalized large and small bowel distension.
6. **Neurogenic** — e.g. spina bifida.

6.40   'Thumbprinting' in the Colon

Colitides

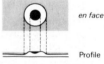

1. **Ulcerative colitis***.
2. **Crohn's disease***.
3. **Ischaemic colitis** — commonest at the splenic flexure, but anywhere possible. Air insufflation may obliterate the 'thumbprinting'.
4. **Pseudomembranous colitis**.
5. **Amoebic colitis**.
6. **Schistosomiasis**.

Neoplastic
1. **Lymphoma***.
2. **Metastases**.

Differential Diagnosis
1. **Pneumatosis coli** — cysts may indent the mucosa, giving a similar appearance, but gas is seen in the wall.

6.41   Aphthoid Ulcers

Barium in a central ulcer surrounded
by a halo of oedematous mucosa.

en face

Profile

In Colon
1. **Crohn's disease*** — the earliest sign in the terminal ileum and colon. Observed in 50% of patients.
2. **Yersinia enterocolitis**.
3. **Amoebic colitis**.
4. **Ischaemic colitis**.
5. **Behçet's disease** — mostly resembles Crohn's disease, but can occasionally simulate an idiopathic ulcerative proctocolitis.

In Small Bowel
1. **Crohn's disease***.
2. **Yersinia enterocolitis**.
3. **Polyarteritis nodosa**.

Further Reading
Simpkins K.C. (1977) Aphthoid ulcers in Crohn's colitis. *Clin. Radiol.*, 28: 601–8.

6.42 Anterior Indentation of the Rectosigmoid Junction

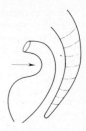

1. **Tumours**
   (a) Peritoneal metastases — common site. Particularly stomach, colon, pancreas and ovary.
   (b) Primary pelvic tumour.
2. **Abscess**.
3. **Haematoma**.
4. **Ascites** — if in erect position.
5. **Endometriosis** — common site.
6. **Hydatid** — metastatic cyst from rupture of a peripheral hepatic cyst.
7. **Surgical** — sling repair for rectal prolapse.

Further Reading

Schulman A. & Fataar S. (1979) Extrinsic stretching, narrowing, and anterior indentation of the rectosigmoid junction. *Clin. Radiol.*, 30: 463–9.

6.43   Widening of the Retrorectal Space

The post-rectal soft-tissue space at
S3–S5 is greater than 1.5 cm.

Normal Variation
40% of cases and these are mostly large or obese individuals.

Inflammatory
1. **Ulcerative colitis*** — seen in 50% of these patients and the
   width increases as the disease progresses.
2. **Crohn's disease*** — the widening may diminish during the
   course of the disease.
3. **Radiotherapy**.
4. **Diverticulitis**.
5. **Abscess**.

Neoplastic
1. **Carcinoma of the rectum**.
2. **Metastases to the rectum** — especially from prostate,
   ovary and bladder.
3. **Sacral tumours** — metastases, plasmacytoma, chordoma
   and, in children, sacrococcygeal teratoma.

Others
1. **Anterior sacral meningocoele** — a sac containing CSF
   protrudes through a round or oval defect in the anterior
   wall of the sacrum. The diagnosis is confirmed by myelography.
2. **Pelvic lipomatosis**.
3. **Enteric duplication cysts**.

Further Reading
Teplick S.K., Stark P., Clark R.E., Metz J.R. and Shapiro J.H. (1978)
    The retrorectal space. *Clin. Radiol.*, 29: 177–84.

Bibliography

General

Bartram C.I. & Kumar P. (1981) *Clinical Radiology in Gastroenterology*. Oxford: Blackwell Scientific Publications.

Laufer I. (1979) *Double Contrast Gastrointestinal Radiology*. Philadelphia: Saunders.

Margulis A.R. & Burhenne H.J. (1983) *Alimentary Tract Roentgenology*, 4th edn. St Louis: Mosby.

Sutton D. (1980) *A Textbook of Radiology and Imaging*, 3rd edn, chaps 32–8. Edinburgh: Churchill Livingstone.

Abdomen

Fataar S. & Schulman A. (1981) Subphrenic abscess: the radiological approach. *Clin. Radiol.*, 32: 147–56.

Felson B. (ed.) (1973) The Acute Abdomen, Part I. Bowel obstruction. *Semin. Roentgenol.*, 8(3)

Felson B. (ed.) (1973) The Acute Abdomen, Part II. Inflammatory disease. *Semin. Roentgenol.*, 8(4).

Meyers M.A. (1981) Intraperitoneal spread of malignancies and its effects on the bowel. *Clin. Radiol.*, 32: 129–46.

Oesophagus

Donner M.W., Saba G.P. & Martinez C.R. (1981) Diffuse diseases of the esophagus: a practical approach. *Semin. Roentgenol.*, 16: 198–213.

Goldstein H.M., Zornoza J. & Hopens T. (1981) Intrinsic disease of the adult oesophagus: benign and malignant tumours. *Semin. Roentgenol.*, 16: 183–97.

Zboralske F.F. & Dodds W.J. (1969) Roentgenographic diagnosis of primary disorders of oesophageal motility. *Radiol. Clin. North Am.*, 7: 147–62.

Stomach

Felson B. (ed.) (1971) Localised lesions of the stomach. *Semin. Roentgenol.*, 6(2).

Ichikawa H. (1973) Differential diagnosis between benign and malignant ulcers of the stomach. *Clin. Gastroenterol.* 2: 329–43.

Small Bowel

Eaton S.B. & Ferrucci J.T. (1973) *Radiology of the Pancreas and Duodenum*. Philadelphia: Saunders.

Marshak R.H. & Lindner A.E. (1976) *Radiology of the Small Intestine*, 2nd edn. Philadelphia: Saunders.

Sellink J.L. (1976) Radiological Atlas of Common Diseases of the Small Bowel. Massachusetts: Stenfert Kroese.
Theoni R.F. & Margulis A.R. (1979) Gastrointestinal tuberculosis. *Semin. Roentgenol.*, 14: 283–94.

Large Bowel
Felson B. (ed.) (1968) Inflammatory diseases of the colon. *Semin. Roentgenol.*, 3(1).
Felson B. (ed.) (1976) Localised solitary lesions of the colon. *Semin. Roentgenol.*, 11(2).
Gardiner R. & Stevenson G.W. (1982) The colitides. *Radiol. Clin. North Am.*, 20: 797–817.
Kolawole T.M. & Lewis E.A. (1974) Radiological observations on intestinal amoebiasis. *Am. J. Roentgenol.*, 122: 257–65.
Wittenberg J., Athanasoulis C.A., Williams L.F., Paredes S., O'Sullivan P. & Brown P. (1975) Ischaemic colitis. *Am. J. Roentgenol.*, 123: 287–300.
Young W.S. (1980) Further radiological observations in caecal volvulus. *Clin. Radiol.*, 31: 479–83.
Young W.S., Engelbrecht H.E. & Stoker A. (1978) Plain film analysis in sigmoid volvulus. *Clin. Radiol.*, 29: 553–60.

Chapter 7
Gallbladder, Liver, Spleen, Pancreas and Adrenals

7.1 Non-visualization of the Gallbladder

During Oral Cholecystography
1. **Technical failures**
   (a) No fatty meal prior to taking of contrast medium.
   (b) Tablets not taken or taken at the wrong time.
   (c) Vomiting or diarrhoea.
   (d) Failure to fast after taking contrast medium.
   (e) Films taken too early or too late.
   (f) Bilirubin greater than 34 mmol.l^{-1}.
2. **Previous cholecystectomy**.
3. **Ectopic gallbladder** — confirmed by taking a film of the entire abdomen.
4. **Cholecystitis**.
5. **Cystic duct obstruction**.

During Intravenous Cholangiography
1. **Technical failures**
   (a) Contrast medium given too rapidly — renal excretion is seen.
   (b) Bilirubin greater than 50 mmol.l^{-1}.
2. **Previous cholecystectomy**.
3. **Ectopic gallbladder**.
4. **Cystic duct obstruction**.
5. **Cholecystitis**.

7.2   Filling Defect in the Gallbladder

Multiple
1. **Calculi** — 30% are radio-opaque. Freely mobile.
2. **Cholesterosis ('strawberry' gallbladder)** — characteristically multiple fixed mural filling defects.

Single and Small
1. **Calculus**.
2. **Adenomyomatosis** — three characteristic signs
   (a) Fundal nodular filling defect.
   (b) Stricture — anywhere in the gallbladder. Sharply
       localized or a diffuse narrowing. More prominent
       following contraction after a fatty meal.
   (c) Rokitansky–Aschoff sinuses — may only be visible
       after gallbladder contraction.

Single and Large
1. **Calculus**.
2. **Carcinoma** — difficult to diagnose as the radiological
   presentation is usually with a non-functioning gallbladder.
   Nearly always associated with gallstones and, therefore, if
   filling does occur it is indistinguishable from them.

7.3 Gas in the Biliary Tract

Irregularly branching gas shadows which do not reach to the liver edge, probably because of the direction of bile flow. The gallbladder may also be outlined.

Within the Bile Ducts
INCOMPETENCE OF THE SPHINCTER OF ODDI
1. **Following sphincterotomy**.
2. **Following passage of a gallstone**.
3. **Patulous sphincter in the elderly**.

POSTOPERATIVE
1. **Cholecystoenterostomy**.
2. **Choledochoenterostomy**.

SPONTANEOUS BILIARY FISTULA
1. **Passage of a gallstone directly from an inflamed gallbladder into the bowel** — 90% of spontaneous fistulae. 57% erode into the duodenum and 18% into the colon. May result in a gallstone ileus.
2. **Duodenal ulcer perforating into the common bile duct** — 6% of spontaneous fistulae.
3. **Malignancy or trauma** — 4% of spontaneous fistulae.

Within the Gallbladder
1. **All of the above**.
2. **Emphysematous cholecystitis** — due to gas-forming organisms and associated with diabetes in 20% of cases. There is intramural and intraluminal gas but, because there is usually cystic duct obstruction, gas is present in the bile ducts in only 20%. The erect film may show an air/bile interface.

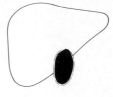

7.4   Gas in the Portal Veins

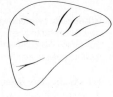

Gas shadows which extend to the periphery of the liver because of the direction of blood flow in the portal veins. Gas may also be present in the portal and mesenteric veins and the bowel wall.

Children

1. **Necrotizing enterocolitis** — 30% develop gas in the portal vein. Necrotic bowel wall allows gas or gas-forming organisms into the portal circulation. The finding of portal vein gas is of grave significance.
2. **Umbilical vein catheterization** — with the inadvertent injection of air.
3. **Erythroblastosis fetalis**.

Adults

1. **Mesenteric infarction** — the majority of patients die soon after gas is seen in the portal veins.
2. **Air embolus during double contrast barium enema** — this has been observed during the examination of severely ulcerated colons and is not associated with a fatal outcome.

Further Reading

Mindelzun R. & McCort J.J. (1980) Hepatic and perihepatic radiolucencies. *Radiol. Clin. North Am.*, 18: 221–38.

Wiot J.F. & Felson B. (1961) Gas in the portal venous system. *Am. J. Roentgenol.*, 86: 920–9.

7.5 Hepatomegaly

Neoplastic
1. **Metastases**.
2. **Hepatoma**.
3. **Lymphoma***.

Raised Venous Pressure
1. **Congestive cardiac failure**.
2. **Constrictive pericarditis**.
3. **Tricuspid stenosis**.
4. **Budd–Chiari syndrome**.

Degenerative
1. **Cirrhosis** — especially alcoholic.
2. **Fatty infiltration**.

Myeloproliferative Disorders
1. **Polycythaemia rubra vera**.
2. **Myelofibrosis**.

Infective
1. **Viral** — infectious and serum hepatitis; infectious mono-nucleosis.
2. **Bacterial** — abscess; brucellosis.
3. **Protozoal** — amoebic abscess, malaria, trypanosomiasis and kala-azar.
4. **Parasitic** — hydatid.

Storage Disorders
1. **Amyloid**.
2. **Haemochromatosis**.
3. **Gaucher's disease**.
4. **Niemann–Pick disease**.

Congenital
1. **Riedel's lobe**.
2. **Polycystic disease***.

7.6   Hepatic Calcification

Multiple and Small
1. **Healed granulomas** — tuberculosis, histoplasmosis and, less commonly, brucellosis and coccidioidomycosis.

Curvilinear
1. **Hydatid** — extensive calcification favours an inactive cyst. Calcification may also be present within the cyst due to calcification of daughter cysts.
2. **Abscess** — especially amoebic abscess when the right lobe is most frequently affected.
3. **(Calcified (porcelain) gallbladder.)**

Localized in a Mass
1. **Metastases** — calcification is uncommon but colloid carcinoma of the rectum, colon or stomach calcify most frequently. It may be amorphous, flakey, stippled or granular and solitary or multiple. Calcification may follow radiotherapy or chemotherapy.
2. **Hepatoma** — rare. Calcifications are punctate, stippled or granular.

Sunray Spiculation
1. **Haemangioma** — phleboliths may also occur but are uncommon.
2. **Metastases** — infrequently in metastases from colloid carcinomas.
3. **Hepatoma**.

Diffuse Increased Density
1. **Haemochromatosis***.
2. **Thorotrast** — lacy, bubbly increased density ± opacification of the liver capsule. Adjacent lymph nodes and spleen also show increased density, although the latter is more granular.

Further Reading
Darlak J.J., Moskowitz M. & Katten K.R. (1980) Calcifications in the liver. *Radiol. Clin. North Am.*, 18: 209–19.

7.7 Splenomegaly

Huge Spleen
1. **Chronic myeloid leukaemia**.
2. **Myelofibrosis**.
3. **Malaria**.
4. **Kala-azar**.
5. **Gaucher's disease**.
6. **Lymphoma***.

Moderately Large Spleen
1. **All of the above**.
2. **Storage diseases**.
3. **Haemolytic anaemias**.
4. **Portal hypertension**.
5. **Leukaemias**.

Slightly Large Spleen
1. **All of the above**.
2. **Infections**
    (a) Viral — infectious hepatitis, infectious mononuc-
        leosis.
    (b) Bacterial — septicaemia, brucellosis, typhoid and
        tuberculosis.
    (c) Rickettsial — typhus.
    (d) Fungal — histoplasmosis.
3. **Sarcoidosis***.
4. **Amyloidosis**.
5. **Rheumatoid arthritis (Felty's syndrome)***.
6. **Systemic lupus erythematosus***.

7.8   Splenic Calcification

Curvilinear
1. **Splenic artery atherosclerosis** — including splenic artery aneurysm.
2. **Cyst** — hydatid or post-traumatic.

Multiple Small Nodular
1. **Phleboliths** — may have small central lucencies.
2. **Haemangioma** — phleboliths.
3. **Tuberculosis**.
4. **Histoplasmosis**.
5. **Brucellosis**.
6. **Sickle-cell anaemia***.

Diffuse Homogeneous or Finely Granular
1. **Sickle-cell anaemia***.
2. **Thorotrast** — densities also in the liver and upper abdominal lymph nodes.

Solitary Greater than 1 cm
1. **Healed infarct or haematoma**.
2. **Healed abscess**.
3. **Tuberculosis**.

Further Reading
McCall I.W., Vaidya S. & Serjeant G.R. (1981) Splenic opacification in homozygous sickle cell disease. *Clin. Radiol.*, 32: 611–15.

7.9 Pancreatic Calcification

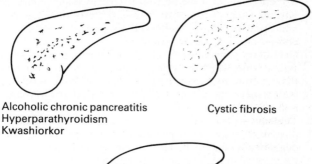

Alcoholic chronic pancreatitis
Hyperparathyroidism
Kwashiorkor

Cystic fibrosis

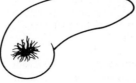

Cystadenocarcinoma

1. **Alcoholic pancreatitis** — calcification, which is almost exclusively due to intraductal calculi, is seen in 20–40% (compared with 2% of gallstone pancreatitis). Usually after 5–10 years of pain. Limited to head or tail in 25%. Rarely solitary. Calculi are numerous, irregular and generally small.

2. **Pseudocyst** — 12–20% exhibit calcification which is usually similar to that seen in chronic pancreatitis but may be curvilinear rim calcification.

3. **Carcinoma of the pancreas** — although for all practical purposes adenocarcinoma does not calcify there is an increased incidence of pancreatic cancer in chronic pancreatitis and the two will be found concurrently in about 2% of cases.

4. **Hyperparathyroidism*** — pancreatitis occurs as a complication of HPT in 10% of cases and 30% of these show calcification which is similar to that observed in chronic pancreatitis. 70% have nephrocalcinosis or urolithiasis and this should suggest the diagnosis.

5. **Cystic fibrosis*** — calcification occurs late in the disease when there is advanced pancreatic fibrosis associated with diabetes mellitus. Calcification is typically finely granular.
6. **Kwashiorkor** — pancreatic lithiasis is a frequent finding and appears before adulthood. Its pattern is similar to chronic alcoholic pancreatitis.
7. **Hereditary pancreatitis** — autosomal dominant. 60% show calcification which is typically rounded and often larger than in other pancreatic diseases. 20% die from pancreatic malignancy. The diagnosis should be considered in young, non-alcoholic patients.
8. **Tumours** — calcification is observed in 10% of cystadenomas and cystadenocarcinomas. It is non-specific but occasionally 'sunburst'. The rare cavernous lymphangioma contains phleboliths in and adjacent to it.
9. **Idiopathic**.

Further Reading

Ring E.J., Eaton S.B., Ferrucci J.T. & Short W.F. (1973) Differential diagnosis of pancreatic calcification. *Am. J. Roentgenol.*, 117: 446–52.

7.10   Adrenal Calcification

Child

1. **Cystic disease** — usually the result of haemorrhage which may be secondary to birth trauma, infection, haemorrhagic disorders or arterial or venous thromboses. Partial or complete ring-like calcification is observed initially but this later becomes compact as the cyst collapses. Frequently asymptomatic.
2. **Neuroblastoma** — in 30–50% of cases. Ill-defined, stippled and non-homogeneous. Lymph-node and liver metastases can also calcify.
3. **Ganglioneuroma** — similar appearance to neuroblastoma, but only 20% are within the adrenal.
4. **Wolman's disease** — a rare autosomal recessive lipoidosis. Hepatomegaly, splenomegaly and adrenomegaly with punctate cortical adrenal calcification is pathognomonic.

Adult

1. **Cystic disease** — similar to that seen in the child. Bilateral in 15% of cases.
2. **Carcinoma** — irregular punctate calcifications. Average size of tumour is 14 cm and there is frequently displacement of the ipsilateral kidney.
3. **Addison's disease** — now most commonly due to autoimmune disease or metastasis. In the past when tuberculosis was a frequent cause calcification was a common finding.
4. **Ganglioneuroma** — 40% occur over the age of 20 years. Slightly flocculent calcifications in a mass which is usually asymptomatic. If the tumour is large enough there will be displacement of the adjacent kidney and/or ureter.
5. **Inflammatory** — primary tuberculosis and histoplasmosis.
6. **Phaeochromocytoma** — calcification is rare but when present is usually an 'eggshell' pattern.

Further Reading

Lecky J.W., Wolfman N.T. & Modic C.W. (1976) Current concepts of adrenal angiography. *Radiol. Clin. North Am.*, 14: 309–52.
Queloz J.M., Capitanio M.A. & Kirkpatrick I.A. (1972) Wolman's disease. Roentgen observations in three siblings. *Radiology*, 104: 357–9.

Chapter 8
Urinary Tract

8.1 Loss of a Renal Outline on the Plain Film

Not necessarily associated with a non-visualized kidney after intravenous contrast medium.

1. **Technical factors** — e.g. poor radiography, overlying faeces, etc.
2. **Congenital absence** — 1:1000 live births. Increased incidence of extrarenal abnormalities (ventricular septal defect, meningomyelocoele, intestinal tract strictures, imperforate anus, skeletal abnormalities and unicornuate uterus). The normal solitary kidney may approach twice normal size.
3. **Displaced or ectopic kidney** — presacral, crossed ectopia or intrathoracic.
4. **Perinephric haematoma** — obliteration of the perirenal fat. ± other signs of trauma, e.g. fractured transverse processes.
5. **Perinephric abscess** — scoliosis concave to the affected side. May be associated with gas in the perirenal tissues. ± localized ileus.
6. **Tumour** — when perinephric fat is replaced by tumour.
7. **Post-nephrectomy** — rare because residual perinephric fat preserves an apparent renal outline. Surgical resection of 12th rib is usually evident.

8.2   Renal Calcification

Calculi (q.v.)

Dystrophic Calcification Due to Localized Disease
Usually one kidney or part of one kidney.

1. **Infections**
    (a) Tuberculosis — variable appearance of nodular, curvilinear or amorphous calcification. Typically multi-focal with calcification elsewhere in the urinary tract.
    (b) Hydatid — curvilinear calcification in the cyst wall.
    (c) Xanthogranulomatous pyelonephritis.
    (d) Abscess.
2. **Carcinoma** — in 6% of carcinomas. Usually amorphous or irregular, but occasionally curvilinear.
3. **Aneurysm** — of the renal artery. Curvilinear.

Nephrocalcinosis
Parenchymal calcification associated with a diffuse renal lesion (i.e. dystrophic calcification) or metabolic abnormality, e.g. hypercalcaemia (metabolic or metastatic calcification). May be medullary or cortical.

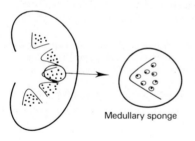

Medullary sponge

Medullary

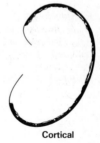

Cortical

MEDULLARY (PYRAMIDAL)
The first three causes account for 70% of cases.
1. **Hyperparathyroidism***.
2. **Renal tubular acidosis** — may be associated with osteo-malacia or rickets. Calcification tends to be more severe than that due to other causes. It is the commonest cause in children.

3. **Medullary sponge kidney** — a variable portion of one or both kidneys contains numerous small medullary cysts which communicate with tubules and therefore opacify during excretion urography. The cysts contain small calculi giving a 'bunch of grapes' appearance. Big kidneys. (Although not strictly a cause of nephrocalcinosis, because it comprises calculi in ectatic ducts, it is included here because of the plain film findings which simulate nephrocalcinosis.)

4. **Renal papillary necrosis** — calcification of necrotic papillae. See section 8.17.

5. **Causes of hypercalcaemia or hypercalciuria**
   (a) Milk alkali syndrome.
   (b) Idiopathic hypercalciuria.
   (c) Sarcoidosis*.
   (d) Hypervitaminosis D.

6. **Oxalosis** — the kidneys may be completely opaque because of diffuse calcification. Presents at a younger age than the other causes of nephrocalcinosis.

CORTICAL

1. **Acute cortical necrosis** — classically 'tramline' calcification.

2. **Chronic glomerulonephritis** — rarely.

3. **Chronic transplant rejection**.

Further Reading

Daniel W.W., Hartman G.W., Witten D.M., Farrow G.M. & Kelalis P.P. (1972) Calcified renal masses. *Radiology*, 103: 503–8.

Lalli A.F. (1982) Renal parenchyma calcifications. *Semin. Roentgenol.*, 17(2): 101–12.

Wrong O.M. & Feest T.G. (1976) Nephrocalcinosis. *Adv. Med.*, 12: 394–406.

8.3 Renal Calculi

Opaque
Calcium phosphate/calcium oxalate, calcium oxalate, calcium phosphate/magnesium ammonium phosphate and calcium phosphate.

Poorly Opaque
Cystine (in cystinuria).

Non-opaque
Uric acid, xanthine and matrix (mucoprotein).

Calcium Containing
1. **With normocalcaemia** — obstruction, urinary tract infection, prolonged bedrest, 'horseshoe' kidney, vesical diverticulum, renal tubular acidosis, medullary sponge kidney and idiopathic hypercalcinuria.
2. **With hypercalcaemia** — hyperparathyroidism, milk–alkali syndrome, excess vitamin D, idiopathic hypercalcaemia of infancy and sarcoidosis.

Pure Calcium Oxalate due to Hyperoxaluria
1. **Hereditary hyperoxaluria** — very rare. Presents in childhood with repeated stones and nephrocalcinosis.
2. **Enteric hyperoxaluria** — due to a disturbance of bile acid metabolism. Mainly in patients with small bowel disease, either Crohn's disease or surgical resection.

Uric Acid
1. **With hyperuricaemia** — gout, myeloproliferative disorders and during the treatment of tumours with antimitotic agents.
2. **With normouricaemia** — idiopathic or associated with acid, concentrated urine (in hot climates and in ileostomy patients).

Xanthine
Due to a failure of normal oxidation of purines.

Matrix
Rare. In poorly functioning, infected urinary tracts.

Further Reading
Banner M.P. & Pollack H.M. (1982) Urolithiasis in the lower urinary tract. *Semin. Roentgenol.*, 17(2): 140–8.
Singh E.O. & Malek R.S. (1982) Calculus disease in the upper urinary tract. *Semin. Roentgenol.*, 17(2): 113–32.
Thornbury J.R. & Parker T.W. (1982) Ureteral calculi. *Semin. Roentgenol.*, 17(2): 133–9.

8.4   Gas in the Urinary Tract

Gas shadows which conform to the position and shape of the bladder, ureters or pelvicalyceal systems.

Gas Inside the Bladder
1. **Vesico-intestinal fistula** — diverticular disease, carcinoma of the colon or rectum and Crohn's disease.
2. **Cystitis** — due to gas-forming organisms and fermentation, especially in diabetics. Usually *Escherichia coli*. Clostridial infections are rare and usually secondary to septicaemia.
3. **Following instrumentation**.
4. **Penetrating wounds**.

Gas in the Bladder Wall
1. **Emphysematous cystitis** — usually in diabetics.

Gas in the Ureters and Pelvicalyceal Systems
1. **Any cause of gas in the bladder**.
2. **Ureteric diversion** — into the colon or bladder.
3. **Fistula** — Crohn's disease or perforated duodenal ulcer.
4. **Infection** — usually in diabetics. Gas may also be present in the renal parenchyma and retroperitoneal tissues.

8.5 Non-visualization of One Kidney During Excretion Urography

1. **Absent kidney** — congenital absence or post-nephrectomy.
2. **Ectopic kidney**.
3. **Chronic obstructive uropathy**.
4. **Infection** — pyonephrosis, xanthogranulomatous pyelo-nephritis or tuberculosis.
5. **Tumour** — an avascular tumour completely replacing the kidney or preventing normal function of residual renal tissue by occluding the renal vein or pelvis.
6. **Renal artery occlusion** — including trauma.
7. **Renal vein occlusion** — see section 8.19.
8. **Multicystic kidney** — see section 8.14.

8.6   Unilateral Small Scarred Kidney

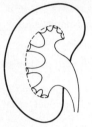

Normal: cortex
parallel to
interpapillary line

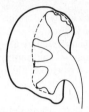

Chronic pyelonephritis

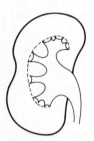

Lobar infarction

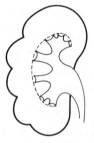

Fetal lobulation

In all these conditions chronic unilateral disease is associated with compensatory hypertrophy of the contralateral kidney.

1. **Chronic pyelonephritis/reflux nephropathy** — a focal scar over a dilated calyx. Usually multifocal and may be bilateral. Scarring is most prominent in the upper and lower poles. Minimal scarring, especially at a pole, produces decreased cortical thickness with a normal papilla and is then indistinguishable from lobar infarction.
2. **Tuberculosis** — calcification differentiates it from the other members of this section.
3. **Lobar infarction** — a broad contour depression over a normal calyx. Normal interpapillary line.

4. **Renal dysplasia** — a forme fruste multicystic kidney. Dilated calyces. Indistinguishable from chronic pyelo-nephritis. Arteriography outlines a small thread-like renal artery.

Differential Diagnosis
1. **Persistent fetal lobulation** — lobules overlie calyces with interlobular septa between the calyces. Normal-size kidney.

Further Reading
Davidson, A.J. (1977) *Radiological Diagnosis of Renal Parenchymal Disease*. chap. 4, pp. 47–68. Philadelphia: Saunders.

8.7 Unilateral Small Smooth Kidney

In all these conditions chronic unilateral disease is associated with compensatory hypertrophy of the contralateral kidney.

With a Dilated Collecting System
1. **Post-obstructive atrophy** — ± thinning of the renal cortex and if there is impaired renal function this will be revealed by poor contrast medium density in the collecting system.

With a Small-volume Collecting System
This is a sign of diminished urinary volume and together with global cortical thinning, delayed opacification of the calyces, increased density of the opacified collecting system and delayed wash-out following oral fluids or diuretics, indicates ischaemia.

1. **Ischaemia due to renal artery stenosis** — ureteric notching is due to enlarged collateral vessels and differentiates this from the other causes in this group. See section 8.18.
2. **Radiation nephritis** — at least 23 Gy (2300 rad) over 5 weeks. The collecting system may be normal or small. Depending on the size of the radiation field both, one or just part of one kidney may be affected. There may be other sequelae of radiotherapy, e.g. scoliosis following radiotherapy in childhood.
3. **End result of renal infarction** — due to previous severe trauma involving the renal artery or renal vein thrombosis. The collecting system does not usually opacify during excretion urography.

With Five or Less Calyces
1. **Congenital hypoplasia** — the pelvicalyceal system is otherwise normal.

Further Reading
Davidson, A.J. (1977) *Radiological Diagnosis of Renal Parenchymal Disease*, chap. 5, pp. 69–95. Philadelphia: Saunders.

8.8   Bilateral Small Smooth Kidneys

1. **Generalized arteriosclerosis** — normal calyces.
2. **Chronic glomerulonephritis** — normal calyces. Reduced nephrogram density and poor calyceal opacification.
3. **Chronic papillary necrosis** (q.v.) — with other signs of necrotic papillae.
4. **Arterial hypotension** — distinguished by the time relationship to the contrast medium injection and its transient nature.
5. **Causes of unilateral small smooth kidneys occurring bilaterally** — e.g. obstructive uropathy or renal artery stenosis.

Further Reading
Davidson, A.J. (1977) *Radiological Diagnosis of Renal Parenchymal Disease*, chap. 6, pp. 96–131. Philadelphia: Saunders.

8.9 Unilateral Large Smooth Kidney

1. **Compensatory hypertrophy**.
2. **Obstructed kidney** dilated calyces.
3. **Pyonephrosis**
4. **Duplex kidney** — female:male, 2:1. Equal incidence on both sides and 20% are bilateral. Incomplete more common than complete. Only 50% are bigger than the contralateral kidney; 40% are the same size; 10% are smaller (Privett et al. 1976).
5. **Tumour** — see section 8.12.
6. **Crossed fused ectopia** — may be associated with anorectal anomalies and renal dysplasia. No kidney on the contra-lateral side and ureter crosses the midline.
7. **Multicystic kidney** — see section 8.14.
8. **Acute pyelonephritis** — impaired excretion of contrast medium. ± increasingly dense nephrogram. Attenuated calyces but may have non-obstructive pelvicalyceal or ureteric dilatation. Completely reversible within a few weeks of clinical recovery.
9. **Trauma** — haematoma or urinoma.
10. **Renal vein thrombosis** — see section 8.19.
11. **Acute arterial infarction**.
12. **Adult polycystic disease*** — asymmetrical bilateral enlargement, but 8% of cases are unilateral. Lobulated rather than completely smooth.

Further Reading

Davidson A.J. (1977) *Radiological Diagnosis of Renal Parenchymal Disease*, chap. 8, pp. 162–92. Philadelphia: Saunders.
Privett J.T.J., Jeans W.D. & Roylance J. (1976) The incidence and importance of renal duplication. *Clin. Radiol.*, 27: 521–30.

8.10   Bilateral Large Smooth Kidneys

It is often difficult to distinguish, radiologically, the members of this group from one another. The appearance of the nephrogram may be helpful — see section 8.16. Associated clinical and radiological abnormalities elsewhere are often more useful, e.g. in sickle-cell anaemia, Goodpasture's disease and acromegaly.

Proliferative and Necrotizing Disorders
1. **Acute glomerulonephritis**.
2. **Polyarteritis nodosa**.
3. **Wegener's granulomatosis**.
4. **Goodpasture's disease**.
5. **Systemic lupus erythematosus***.

Deposition of Abnormal Proteins
1. **Amyloid** — renal involvement in 80% of secondary and 35% of primary amyloid. Chronic deposition results in small kidneys.
2. **Multiple myeloma***.

Abnormal Fluid Accumulation
1. **Acute tubular necrosis**.
2. **Acute cortical necrosis** — may show an opacified medulla and outer rim with non-opacified cortex. Cortical calcification is a late finding.

Neoplastic Infiltration
1 **Leukaemia and lymphoma**.

Inflammatory Cell Infiltration
1. **Acute interstitial nephritis**.

Miscellaneous
1. **Renal vein thrombosis** (q.v.).
2. **Acute renal papillary necrosis** (q.v.).
3. **Polycystic disease*** — infantile form has smooth outlines.
4. **Acute urate nephropathy**.
5. **Sickle-cell anaemia***.
6. **Bilateral hydronephrosis**.
7. **Medullary sponge kidneys** — with 'bunch of grapes' calcification.
8. **Acromegaly* and gigantism** — as part of the generalized visceromegaly.

Further Reading
Davidson, A.J. (1977) *Radiological Diagnosis of Renal Parenchymal Disease*, chap. 7, pp. 132–61. Philadelphia: Saunders.

8.11 Localized Bulge of the Renal Outline

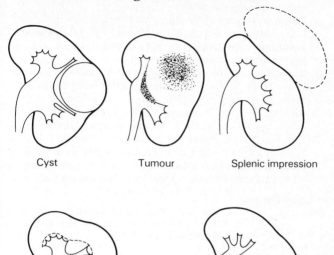

Cyst

Tumour

Splenic impression

Dromedary hump

Enlarged column
of Bertin

1. **Cyst** — well defined nephrographic defect with a thin wall on the outer margin. Beak sign. Displacement and distortion of smooth-walled calyces without obliteration.
2. **Tumour** — mostly renal cell carcinoma in adults and Wilms' tumour in children. See section 8.12.
3. **Fetal lobulation** — the lobule directly overlies a normal calyx. Normal interpapillary line. See section 8.6.
4. **Dromedary hump** — on the mid portion of the lateral border of the kidney. The arc of the interpapillary line parallels the renal contour.

5. **Splenic impression** — on the left side only. This produces an apparent bulge inferiorly.
6. **Enlarged column of Bertin** — most commonly in duplication or attempted duplication. Normal ^{99}Tc-DMSA scan.
7. **Localized hypertrophy** — e.g. adjacent to an area of pyelonephritic scarring.
8. **Abscess** — loss of renal outline and psoas margin on the control film. Scoliosis concave to the involved side. Initially there is no nephrographic defect but following central necrosis there will be a central defect surrounded by a thick irregular wall. Adjacent calyces are displaced or effaced.
9. **Non-functioning moiety of a duplex** — usually a hydronephrotic upper moiety. Delayed films may show contrast medium in the upper moiety calyces. Lower moiety calyces have 'drooping flowers' appearance. See section 8.22.

Further Reading

Felson B. & Moskowitz M. (1969) Renal pseudotumours. The regenerated nodule and other lumps, bumps and dromedary humps. *Am. J. Roentgenol.*, 107: 720–9.

8.12   Renal Neoplasms

Malignant

1. **Renal cell carcinoma** — 90% of adult malignant tumours. Bilateral in 10% and an increased incidence of bilaterality in polycystic kidneys and von Hippel–Lindau disease. A mass lesion (showing irregular or amorphous calcification in 10% of cases). Calyces are obliterated, distorted and/or displaced. Half-shadow filling defect in a calyx or pelvis. Arteriography shows a typical pathological circulation in the majority.
2. **Transitional cell carcinoma** — usually papilliferous. May obstruct or obliterate a calyx or obstruct a whole kidney. Seeding may produce a second lesion further down the urinary tract. Bilateral tumours are rare. Calcification in 2%.
3. **Squamous cell carcinoma** — ulcerated plaque or stricture. 50% are associated with calculi. There is usually a large parenchymal mass before there is any sizeable intrapelvic mass. No calcification. Avascular at arteriography.

4. **Wilms' tumour** — 80% present in the first 3 years. Bilateral in 5%. Increased incidence with aniridia, hemihypertrophy and 'horseshoe' kidney. Can be familial. Radiological signs similar to renal cell carcinoma. Streaky and amorphous calcification in 5%. Mesoblastic nephroma is urographically indistinguishable from Wilms' tumour but occurs in very young infants. It does not metastasize and complete excision results in cure.

5. **Leukaemia/lymphoma** — bilateral large smooth kidneys. Thickened parenchyma with compression of the pelvicalyceal systems.

6. **Metastases** — not uncommon. Usually multiple. Bronchus, breast and stomach.

Benign

1. **Hamartoma** — usually solitary but often multiple and bilateral in tuberous sclerosis. Diagnostic appearance on the plain film of radiolucent fat (but only observed in 9%). Other signs are of any mass lesion and angiography does not differentiate from renal cell carcinoma.

2. **Adenoma** — usually small and frequently multiple. Majority are found at autopsy. Hypovascular at arteriography.

3. **Others** — myoma, lipoma, haemangioma and fibroma are all rare.

Further Reading
See end of chapter.

8.13   Classification of Renal Cysts

(After Elkin & Bernstein, 1969.)

Renal Dysplasia
1. **Multicystic kidney** — see section 8.14.
2. **Focal and segmental cystic dysplasia.**
3. **Multiple cysts associated with lower urinary tract obstruction.**

*Polycystic Disease**
1. **Infantile polycystic disease**
   (a) Polycystic disease of the newborn.
   (b) Polycystic disease of childhood.
2. **Adult polycystic disease**.

Cortical Cysts
1. **Trisomy 13 and 18** — numerous small cysts producing no functional disturbance.
2. **Tuberous sclerosis*** — usually small but may be large and the condition is progressive.
3. **Simple cyst** — unilocular. Increase in size and number with age.
4. **Multilocular cyst** — rare. Unilateral. Appearance is otherwise similar to a simple cyst. 50% occur in children less than 5 years of age.

Medullary Cysts
1. **Medullary sponge kidney** — bilateral in 60–80%. Multiple, small, mainly pyramidal cysts which opacify during excretion urography and contain calculi.
2. **Medullary cystic disease** — rare. Multiple cysts result in a 'honeycomb' pattern with sparing of the cortex. Progressive renal failure.
3. **Papillary necrosis** — see section 8.17.
4. **Pyelogenic (calyceal) cyst** — small, usually solitary cyst communicating via an isthmus with the fornix of a calyx.

Miscellaneous Intrarenal Cysts
1. **Inflammatory**
    (a) Tuberculosis.
    (b) Calculus disease.
    (c) Hydatid.
2. **Neoplastic** — cystic degeneration of a carcinoma.
3. **Traumatic** — intrarenal haematoma.

Extraparenchymal Renal Cysts
1. **Parapelvic cyst** — located in or near the hilum, but does not communicate with the renal pelvis and therefore does not opacify during urography. Simple or multilocular; single or multiple; unilateral or bilateral. It compresses the renal pelvis and may cause hydronephrosis.
2. **Perinephric cyst** — beneath the capsule or between the capsule and perinephric fat. Secondary to trauma, obstruction or replacement of haematoma. It may compress the kidney, pelvis or ureter, leading to hydronephrosis or causing displacement of the kidney.

Further Reading

Elkin M. & Bernstein J. (1969) Cystic diseases of the kidney — radiological and pathological considerations. *Clin. Radiol.*, 20: 65–82.
Madewell J.E., Hartman D.S. & Lichtenstein J.E. (1979) Radiologic--pathologic correlations in cystic disease of the kidney. *Radiol. Clin. North Am.*, 17: 261–79.

8.14   Renal Mass in the Newborn and Young Infant

1. **Hydronephrosis** (q.v.) — uni- or bilateral.
2. **Multicystic kidney** — unilateral, but 30% have an abnormal contralateral kidney (mostly pelviureteric junction obstruction). Non-functioning, multilobulated kidney. Rarely, nephrographic crescents and late pooling of contrast medium in cysts is observed. Curvilinear calcification is characteristic but only seen occasionally. Ultrasound reveals multiple cysts of unequal size. The commonest renal mass in the first year of life.
3. **Polycystic kidneys** (see Polycystic disease*) — bilateral. Poor renal excretion. Striated nephrogram with no visualization of calyces.
4. **Renal vein thrombosis** (q.v.) — uni- or bilateral.
5. **Nephroblastoma or mesoblastic nephroma** — see section 8.12. Unilateral. No nephrographic defect. Deformed or replaced calyces.
6. **Renal ectopia**.

8.15   Hydronephrosis in a Child

1. **Pelviureteric junction obstruction** — more common on the left side. 20% bilateral. Due to stricture, neuromuscular inco-ordination, aberrant vessels or atresia. Contralateral kidney is dysplastic in 25% of cases and absent in 12%.
2. **Bladder outflow obstruction** (q.v.) — bilateral upper tract dilatation.
3. **Ureterovesical obstruction** — more common in males and more common on the left side. May be bilateral.
4. **Reflux without obstruction**.
5. **Associated with urinary tract infection** — but no obstruction or reflux. ? represents atony.
6. **Neurogenic**.

Further Reading
Lebowitz R.L. & Griscom N.T. (1977) Neonatal hydronephrosis: 146 cases. *Radiol. Clin. North Am.*, 15: 49–59.

8.16 Nephrographic Patterns

Immediate Faint Persistent Nephrogram
1. **Proliferative/necrotizing disorders** — e.g. acute glomeru-lonephritis. See section 8.10.
2. **Renal vein thrombosis.**
3. **Chronic severe ischaemia.**

Immediate Distinct Persistent Nephrogram
1. **Acute tubular necrosis** — in 60% of cases.
2. **Other causes of acute renal failure.**
3. **Acute-on-chronic renal failure.**
4. **Acute hypotension** — uncommonly.

Increasingly Dense Nephrogram
1. **Acute obstruction** — including urate nephropathy.
2. **Acute hypotension.**
3. **Acute tubular necrosis** — in 30% of cases.
4. **Acute pyelonephritis.**
5. **Multiple myeloma.**
6. **Renal vein thrombosis.**
7. **Acute glomerulonephritis.**
8. **Amyloid.**
9. **Acute papillary necrosis** — and rarely chronic papillary necrosis.

Rim Nephrogram
1. **Severe hydronephrosis** — scalloped nephrogram with a negative pyelogram.
2. **Acute complete arterial occlusion** — smooth nephrogram from cortical perfusion by capsular arteries.

Striated Nephrogram
1. **Acute ureteric obstruction.**
2. **Infantile polycystic disease** — contrast medium in dilated tubules.
3. **Medullary sponge kidney** — in the medulla only. Parallel or fan-shaped streaks radiating from the papilla to the periphery of the kidney.
4. **Acute pyelonephritis.**

Further Reading
Newhouse, J.H. & Pfister, R.C. (1979) The nephrogram. *Radiol. Clin. North Am.*, 17: 213–26.

8.17   Renal Papillary Necrosis

1. Normal — small kidneys with smooth outlines.
2. Bilateral in 85% with multiple papillae affected.
3. Papillae may show
   (a) Enlargement (early).
   (b) Partial sloughing — a fissure forms and may communicate with a central irregular cavity.
   (c) Total sloughing — the sloughed papillary tissue may (i) fragment and be passed in the urine, (ii) cause ureteric obstruction, (iii) remain free in a calyx, or (iv) remain in the pelvis and form a ball calculus.
   (d) Necrosis-in-situ — the papilla is shrunken and necrotic but has not separated.
4. Calyces will appear dilated following total sloughing of a papilla.
5. Calcification and occasionally ossification of a shrunken, necrotic papilla. If marginal, it appears as a calculus with a radiolucent centre.

Normal   Swollen   Partial papillary necrosis   Total papillary necrosis   Necrosis-in-situ

A useful mnemonic is *ADIPOSE*—

A Analgesics — phenacetin and aspirin
D Diabetes
I Infants in shock
P Pyelonephritis
O Obstruction
S Sickle cell disease
E Ethanol.

However, diabetes, analgesics and sickle-cell anaemia are the most important, with diabetes the most frequent cause.

Further Reading

Hare W.S.C. and Poynter J.D. (1974) The radiology of renal papillary necrosis as seen in analgesic nephropathy. *Clin. Radiol.*, 25: 423–43.

8.18 Renal Induced Hypertension

Signs of Unilateral Renal Artery Stenosis
1. Unilateral delay of 1 minute or more in the appearance of opacified calyces.
2. Small, smooth kidney
   — left more than 1.5 cm shorter than the right
   — right more than 2 cm shorter than the left.
3. Increased density of opacified calyces.
4. Ureteric notching by collateral vessels.

Renal Artery
1. **Arteriosclerosis** — 66% of renovascular causes. Stenosis of the proximal 2 cm of the renal artery; less frequently the distal artery or early branches at bifurcations. More common in males.
2. **Fibromuscular dysplasia** — 33% of renovascular causes. Stenoses ± dilatations which may give the characteristic 'string of beads' appearance. Mainly females less than 40 years. Bilateral in 60% of cases.
3. **Thrombosis/embolism**.
4. **Arteritis** — polyarteritis nodosa, thromboangiitis obliterans, Takayasu's disease, syphilis, congenital rubella or idiopathic.
5. **Neurofibromatosis*** — ± coarctation of the aorta. ± stenoses of other arteries. ± intrarenal arterial abnormalities.
6. **Trauma**.
7. **Aneurysm** — of the aorta or the renal artery.
8. **Arteriovenous fistula** — traumatic, congenital or a stump fistula following nephrectomy.
9. **Extrinsic compression** — neoplasm, aneurysm or lymph nodes.

Chronic Bilateral Parenchymal Disease
1. **Chronic glomerulonephritis**.
2. **Chronic pyelonephritis**.
3. **Adult polycystic disease***.
4. **Diabetic glomerulosclerosis**.
5. **Connective tissue disorders** — systemic lupus erythematosus, scleroderma and polyarthritis nodosa.
6. **Radiotherapy**.
7. **Hydronephrosis**.

8. **Analgesic nephropathy**.
9. **Renal vein thrombosis**.

Unilateral Parenchymal Disease
Much less common as a cause of hypertension.

1. **Chronic pyelonephritis**.
2. **Hydronephrosis**.
3. **Tumours** — hypertension is more common with Wilms' tumour than with renal cell carcinoma. The rare juxta-glomerular cell tumour secretes renin.
4. **Tuberculosis**.
5. **Xanthogranulomatous pyelonephritis**.
6. **Radiotherapy**.
7. **Renal vein thrombosis**.

Further Reading
Webb J.A.W. & Talner L.B. (1979) The role of intravenous urography in hypertension. *Radiol. Clin. North Am.* , 17: 187–95.

8.19   Renal Vein Thrombosis

Unilateral or bilateral.

Sudden —
1. Large non-functioning kidney which over a period of several months becomes small and atrophic.
2. Retrograde pyelography reveals thickened parenchyma (due to oedema) with elongation and compression of the major calyces.
3. Arteriography shows stretching and separation of arterial branches with decreased flow and a poor persistent nephrogram. No opacification of the renal vein.

Gradual —
1. Large kidney.
2. Nephrogram may be normal, poor persistent or increasingly dense.
3. Thickened parenchyma with elongation of major calyces.
4. Ureteric notching due to venous collaterals.

Children
1. **Dehydration and shock** — especially infants delivered of diabetic mothers.
2. **Nephrotic syndrome**.
3. **Cyanotic heart disease**.

Adults
1. **Extension of renal cell carcinoma into the renal vein**.
2. **Local compression by tumour or retroperitoneal nodes**.
3. **Extension of thrombus from the inferior vena cava**.
4. **Trauma**.
5. **Secondary to renal disease** — especially amyloid and chronic glomerulonephritis with nephrotic syndrome.

8.20 Radiolucent Filling Defect in the Renal Pelvis or a Calyx

Technical Factors
1. **Incomplete filling during excretion urography**.
2. **Overlying gas shadows**.

Extrinsic with a Smooth Margin
1. **Cyst** (q.v.).
2. **Vascular impression** — an intrarenal artery producing linear transverse or oblique compression lines and most commonly indenting an upper pole calyx, especially on the right side.
3. **Renal sinus lipomatosis** — most commonly in older patients with a wasting disease of the kidney. Fat in the renal hilum produces a relative lucency and narrows and elongates the major calyces.
4. **Collateral vessels** — most commonly ureteric artery collaterals in renal artery stenosis. Multiple small irregularities in the pelvic wall.

Inseparable from the Wall and with Smooth Margins
1. **Blood clot** — due to trauma, tumour or bleeding diathesis. May be adherent to the wall or free in the lumen. Change in size or shape over several days.
2. **Papilloma** — solitary or multiple.
3. **Pyeloureteritis cystica** — due to chronic infection. Multiple well-defined submucosal cysts project into the lumen of the pelvis and/or ureter.

Arising from the Wall with an Irregular Margin
1. **Transitional cell carcinoma** ⎤
2. **Squamous cell carcinoma** ⎬ see section 8.12.
3. **Renal cell carcinoma** ⎦
4. **Squamous metaplasia (cholesteatoma)** — occurs rarely in association with chronic irritation from a calculus. Indistinguishable from tumour and may be premalignant.

In the Lumen
1. **Blood clot**.
2. **Lucent calculus** (q.v.).
3. **Sloughed papilla**.
4. **Air** (q.v.).

Further Reading
Brown R.C., Jones M.C., Boldus R. & Flocks R.H. (1973) Lesions causing radiolucent defects in the renal pelvis. *Am. J. Roentgenol.*, 119: 770–8.

8.21   Dilated Calyx

With a Narrow Infundibulum
1. **Stricture** — tumour, calculus or tuberculosis.
2. **Extrinsic impression by an artery** — most commonly a right upper pole calyx.
3. **Hydrocalycosis** — may be a congenital anomaly. Can only be safely diagnosed in childhood when calculus, tumour and tuberculosis are uncommon.

With a Wide Infundibulum
1. **Post-obstructive atrophy** — generally all the calyces are affected and associated with parenchymal thinning.
2. **Megacalyces** — dilated calyces ± a slightly dilated pelvis. ± stones. Increased number of calyces — 20–25 (normal 8–12). Because of the large volume collecting system full visualization during urography is delayed. Normal cortical thickness and good renal function differentiate it from post obstructive atrophy.
3. **Polycalycosis** — rare. ± ureteric abnormalities.

Further Reading
Talner L.B. & Gittes R.F. (1974) Megacalyces, further observations and differentiation from obstructive renal disease. *Am. J. Roentgenol.*, 121: 473–86.

8.22   Non-visualization of a Calyx

1. **Technical factors** — incomplete filling during excretion urography.
2. **Tumour** — most commonly a renal cell carcinoma (adult) or Wilms' tumour (child).
3. **Obstructed infundibulum** — due to tumour, calculus or tuberculosis.
4. **Duplex kidney** — with a non-functioning upper or lower moiety. Signs suggesting a non-functioning upper moiety are
   (a) Fewer calyces than the contralateral kidney. This sign is only reliable in unilateral duplication. (Calyceal distribution is symmetrical in 80% of normal individuals.)
   (b) A shortened upper calyx which does not reach into the upper pole.
   (c) The upper calyx of the lower moiety may be deformed by a dilated upper pole pelvis.
   (d) The kidney may be displaced downward by a dilated upper moiety pelvis. The appearances mimic a space occupying lesion in the upper pole.
   (e) The upper pole may be rotated laterally and downward by a dilated upper moiety pelvis and the lower pole calyces adopt a 'drooping flower' appearance.
   (f) Lateral displacement of the entire kidney by a dilated upper moiety ureter.
   (g) The lower moiety ureter may be displaced or compressed by the upper pole ureter, resulting in a series of scalloped curves.
   (h) The lower moiety renal pelvis may be displaced laterally and its ureter then takes a direct oblique course to the lumbosacral junction.
5. **Infection** — abscess or tuberculosis.
6. **Partial nephrectomy** — with a surgical defect in the 12th rib.

8.23 Dilated Ureter

Obstruction

WITHIN THE LUMEN

1. **Calculus** (q.v.).
2. **Blood clot**.
3. **Sloughed papilla**.

IN THE WALL

1. **Oedema or stricture due to calculus**.
2. **Tumour** — carcinoma or papilloma.
3. **Tuberculous stricture** — a particular hazard during the early weeks of treatment.
4. **Schistosomiasis** — especially the distal ureter. ± calcification in the ureter or bladder.
5. **Post surgical trauma** — e.g. a misplaced ligature.
6. **Ureterocoele**.
7. **Megaureter** — symmetrical tapered narrowing above the uretero-vesical junction.

OUTSIDE THE WALL

1. **Retroperitoneal fibrosis** (q.v.).
2. **Carcinoma of cervix, bladder or prostate**.
3. **Retrocaval ureter** — right side only. Distal ureter lies medial to the dilated proximal portion.

Vesico-ureteric Reflux

No Obstruction or Reflux

1. **Post partum** — more common on the right side.
2. **Following relief of obstruction** — most commonly calculus or prostatectomy.
3. **Urinary tract infection**.

8.24   Retroperitoneal Fibrosis

1. Ureteric obstruction of variable severity. 75% bilateral.
2. Tapering lumen or complete obstruction — usually at L4–5 level and never the extreme lower end.
3. Medial deviation of the ureters — more significant if there is a right-angled step in the ureter rather than a gentle drift.

1. **Retroperitoneal malignancy** — lymphoma and metastases from colon and breast especially. The tumour initiates a fibrotic reaction around itself.
2. **Inflammatory conditions** — Crohn's disease, diverticular disease, actinomycosis, pancreatitis and extravasation of urine from the pelvicalyceal system.
3. **Aortic aneurysm** ⎫ fibrosis occurs secondary to blood
4. **Trauma**   ⎬ in the retroperitoneal tissues.
5. **Surgery**   ⎭
6. **Drugs** — methysergide.
7. **Idiopathic**.

Differential Diagnosis of Medially Placed Ureters
1. **Pelvic lipomatosis** — other signs suggesting the diagnosis are (a) elevation and elongation of the bladder, (b) elongation of the rectum and sigmoid with widening of the retrorectal space, and (c) increased lucency of the pelvic wall.
2. **Following abdomino-perineal resection** — the ureters are medially placed inferiorly.
3. **Retrocaval ureter** — the right ureter passes behind the inferior vena cava at the level of LV4. The distal ureter lies medial to the dilated proximal portion.
4. **Normal variant**.

8.25   Filling Defect in the Bladder (in the Wall or in the Lumen)

1. **Prostate.**
2. **Neoplasm** — especially transitional cell carcinoma in an adult and rhabdomyosarcoma in a child.
3. **Blood clot.**
4. **Instrument** — urethral or suprapubic catheter.
5. **Calculus.**
6. **Ureterocoele.**
7. **Schistosomiasis.**
8. **Endometriosis.**

8.26   Bladder Calcification

In the Lumen
1. **Calculus.**
2. **Foreign body** — encrusted.

In the Wall
1. **Transitional cell carcinoma** — surface calcification.
2. **Schistosomiasis.**
3. **Tuberculosis.**

8.27   Bladder Fistula

1. **Crohn's disease***.
2. **Diverticular disease.**
3. **Carcinoma of colon, bladder or reproductive organs.**
4. **Anal atresia** — the majority have fistulae to the bladder, urethra, vagina or perineum.
5. **Postoperative.**
6. **Radiotherapy.**
7. **Trauma.**

8.28   Bladder Outflow Obstruction in a Child

1. Distended bladder with incomplete emptying.
2. ± bilateral upper tract dilatation.
3. ± upper tract cystic disease.

Causes (from proximal to distal)

1. **Vesical diverticulum** — posteriorly behind the bladder base. It fills during micturition and compresses the bladder neck and proximal urethra. More common in males.
2. (**Bladder neck obstruction** — probably not a distinct entity and only occurs as part of other problems such as ectopic ureterocoele and rhabdomyosarcoma.)
3. **Ectopic ureterocoele** — 80% are associated with the upper moiety of a duplex kidney. 15% are bilateral. More common in females. Opens into the urethra, bladder neck or vestibule. May be largely outside the bladder and the bladder base may be elevated. 'Drooping flower' appearance of lower moiety. May prolapse into the urethra.
4. **Posterior urethral valves** — posterior urethra is dilated and the distal urethra is small. Almost exclusively males.
5. **Anterior urethral diverticulum (valve)** — lies inferiorly and the distal mucosal lip obstructs flow. In females the majority are congenital, whilst in males the majority are secondary to periurethral abscess or trauma.
6. **Urethral stricture**.
7. **Prune-belly syndrome** — almost exclusively males. High mortality. Bilateral hydronephrosis and hydroureters with a distended bladder are associated with undescended testes, agenesis of the anterior abdominal wall and urethral obstruction.
8. **Calculus or foreign body**.
9. **Meatal stenosis** } clinical diagnosis.
10. **Phimosis**

N.B. The commonest cause in males is posterior urethral valves and in females is ectopic ureterocoele.

8.29   Calcification of the Seminal Vesicles or Vas Deferens

1. **Diabetes mellitus** — the cause in the vast majority of cases.
2. **Chronic infection** — tuberculosis, schistosomiasis, chronic urinary tract infection and syphilis.
3. **Idiopathic**.

Further Reading
King J.C. & Rosenbaum H.D. (1971) Calcification of the vasa deferentia in non-diabetics. *Radiology*, 100: 603–6.

Bibliography

General
Chrispin A.R., Gordon I., Hall C. & Metreweli C. (1980) *Diagnostic Imaging of the Kidney and Urinary Tract in Children*. Berlin: Springer International.
Davidson A.J. (1977) *Radiological Diagnosis of Renal Parenchymal Disease*. Philadelphia: Saunders.
Davidson A.J. (ed.) (1979) Advances in uroradiology. *Radiol. Clin. North Am.*, 17(2).
Sherwood T. (1980) *Uroradiology*. Oxford: Blackwell.
Sutton D. (ed.) (1980) *Textbook of Radiology and Imaging*, 3rd edn, chaps 39–46. Edinburgh: Churchill Livingstone.
Witten D.M., Myers G.H. & Utz D.C. (1977) *Clinical Urography*, 4th edn. Philadephia: Saunders.

Infections
Felson B. (ed.) (1971) Infections of the urinary tract. *Semin. Roentgenol.*, 6(3).
Gingell J.C., Roylance J., Davies E.R. & Penry J.B. (1973) Xanthogranulomatous pyelonephritis, *Br. J. Radiol.*, 46: 99–109.
Kirkland K. (1966) Urological aspects of hydatid disease, *Br. J. Urol.*, 38: 241–54.
Roylance J., Penry J. B., Davies E.R. & Roberts M. (1970) The radiology of tuberculosis of the urinary tract. *Clin. Radiol.*, 21: 163–70.
Silver T.M., Kass E.J. Thornbury J.R., Konnack J.W. & Wolfman M.G. (1976) The radiological spectrum of acute pyelonephritis in adults and adolescents. *Radiology*, 118: 65–71.
Tonkin A.K. & Whitten D.M. (1979) Genitourinary tuberculosis, *Semin. Roentgenol.*, 14: 305–18.

Watt I. & Roylance J. (1975) Pyonephrosis, *Clin. Radiol.*, 27: 513–19.

Neoplasms

Bruneton J.N., Ballanger P., Ballanger R. & Delorme G. (1979) Renal adenomas. *Clin. Radiol.*, 30: 343–52.

Cope J.R., Roylance J. & Gordon I.R.S. (1972) The radiological features of Wilms' tumours. *Clin. Radiol.*, 23: 331–9.

Lowe P.P. & Roylance J. (1976) Transitional cell carcinoma of the kidney. *Clin. Radiol.*, 27: 503–12.

Martinez-Maldonado M. & Ramirez de Arellano G.A. (1966) Renal involvement in malignant lymphomas. *J. Urol.*, 95: 485–8.

McCallum R.W. (1975) The preoperative diagnosis of renal hamartoma. *Clin. Radiol.*, 26: 257–60.

Thomas J.L., Barnes P.A., Bernardino M.E. & Lewis E. (1982) Diagnostic approaches to adrenal and renal metastases. *Radiol. Clin. North Am.*, 20: 531–44.

Chapter 9
Soft Tissues

9.1 Gynaecomastia

Physiological
1. **Neonatal** — due to high placental oestrogens.
2. **Pubertal** — due to an excess of oestradiol over testosterone.
3. **Senile** — due to falling androgen and rising oestrogen levels with age.

Pharmacological
1. **Oestrogen** — especially in the treatment of carcinoma of the prostate.
2. **Digitalis** — binds to oestrogen receptors.
3. **Anti-cancer drugs** — producing testicular damage.
4. **Anti-androgens** — spironolactone.
5. **Reserpine**.
6. **Phenothiazines**.
7. **Tricyclic antidepressants**.
8. **Methyldopa**.

Pathological
1. **Carcinoma of the bronchus** ⎫ secreting human chorionic
2. **Teratoma of the testis** ⎭ gonadotrophin.
3. **Cirrhosis** — due to increased conversion of androgens to oestrogens.
4. **Hypogonadism** — e.g. Klinefelter's syndrome and castration.
5. **Hypopituitarism** — including acromegaly.
6. **Testicular feminization** — androgen insensitivity.
7. **Adrenal tumours** ⎫ secreting oestrogens.
8. **Leydig cell tumours** ⎭

9.2   Linear and Curvilinear Calcification in Soft Tissues

Arterial
1. **Atheroma/aneurysm**.
2. **Diabetes**.
3. **Hyperparathyroidism*** — more common in secondary than primary.
4. **Werner's syndrome** — premature ageing in a Jewish diabetic (male or female).

Nerve
1. **Leprosy**.
2. **Neurofibromatosis***.

Ligament
1. **Tendinitis** — Pellegrini–Stieda syndrome, supraspinatus.
2. **Ankylosing spondylitis***.
3. **Fluorosis**.
4. **Diabetes**.
5. **Alkaptonuria**.

Bismuth Injection — in the buttocks. ± neuropathic joints.

Parasites
1. ***Cysticerci***   — oval with lucent centre. Often arranged in the direction of muscle fibres.

2. **Guinea worm**   — irregular coiled appearance.

3. *Loa loa*   — thread-like coil. Particularly in the web spaces of the hand.

4. *Armillifer*   — 'comma' shaped. Only in trunk muscles.

See also section 9.4.

9.3   Conglomerate Calcification in Soft Tissues

Collagenoses
1. **Scleroderma*** — acrolysis and flexion contractures in the hands.
2. **Dermatomyositis**.
3. **Ehlers–Danlos syndrome**.

Metabolic
1. **Hyperparathyroidism*** — more common in secondary hyperparathyroidism. Vascular calcification is common.
2. **Gout*** — calcified tophus.

Traumatic
1. **Haematoma**.
2. **Burns**.
3. **Myositis ossificans** — outer part is more densely calcified than the centre.

Infective
1. **Tuberculous abscess/node**.

Neoplastic
1. **Benign**
   (a) Parosteal lipoma — lucent. ± pressure erosion of adjacent bone.
   (b) Haemangioma — Suspect if phleboliths present in an unusual site. ± soft-tissue mass with adjacent bone destruction.
2. **Malignant**
   (a) Parosteal osteosarcoma — age 20–40. Lobulated calcification around a metaphysis. Inner part is more densely calcified than the periphery. Early — a thin lucent line may separate it from underlying bone.
   (b) Juxta-cortical chondrosarcoma — particularly pelvis.
   (c) Liposarcoma.

9.4 'Sheets' of Calcification/Ossification in Soft Tissues

1. **Congenital myositis ossificans progressiva** — manifest in childhood. Initially neck and trunk muscles involved. Short first metacarpal and metatarsal.
2. **Dermatomyositis**.

9.5 Periarticular Soft-tissue Calcification

Inflammatory
1. **Scleroderma*** — ± acro-osteolysis.
2. **Dermatomyositis**.
3. **Gout*** — calcified tophi. Punched-out erosions.
4. **Bursitis** — can be dense and lobulated.

Degenerative
1. **Calcific periarthritis (calcium hydroxyapatite deposition disease)**.
2. **Calcium pyrophosphate deposition disease***.

Renal Failure
1. **Secondary hyperparathyroidism** — ± vascular calcification.
2. **Treatment with 1-α-OHD$_3$** — particularly shoulder, hip and metacarpophalangeal joints.

Hypercalcaemia
1. **Sarcoidosis*** — rare. Affects hands and feet. ± lace-like trabecular pattern in tubular bones.
2. **Hypervitaminosis D**.
3. **Milk–alkali syndrome**.

Neoplastic
1. **Synovial osteochondromatosis** — age 20–50 years. Most commonly affects a large joint. Multiple calcified loose bodies. ± secondary degenerative changes or pressure erosion of bone.
2. **Synovioma** — age 20–50 years. Soft-tissue mass with amorphous calcification, irregular bone destruction and osteoporosis.

Idiopathic
1. **Tumoral calcinosis** — age 20–30 years. Adjacent to a major joint. Firm, non-tender, moveable mass which is well defined, lobulated and calcified on X-ray. Osseous involvement is rare. ± calcium fluid level.

9.6   Soft-tissue Ossification

Traumatic
1. **Myositis ossificans**.
2. **Burns**.
3. **Paraplegia** — ossification adjacent to the ischium — may be related to pressure sores.

Neoplastic
1. **Parosteal osteosarcoma**.
2. **Liposarcoma**.

Congenital Myositis Ossificans Progressiva

9.7   Increased Heel Pad Thickness

males: if 'x' is greater than 23 mm.
females: if 'x' is greater than 21.5 mm.

1. **Acromegaly***.
2. **Obesity**.
3. **Peripheral oedema**.
4. **Infection/injury**.
5. **Myxoedema**.
6. **Epanutin therapy**.

Further Reading
Kattan K.R. (1975) Thickening of the heel pad associated with long-term Dilantin therapy. *Am. J. Roentgenol.*, 124: 52–6.
Kho K.M., Wright A.D. & Doyle F.H. (1970) Heel pad thickness in acromegaly. *Br. J. Radiol.*, 43: 119–22.

Bibliography

Cockshott P. & Middlemiss J.H. (1979) *Clinical Radiology in the Tropics*. Edinburgh: Churchill Livingstone.
Griffiths H.J. (1976) *Radiology of Renal Failure*. Philadelphia: Saunders.
Palmer P.E.S. (1966) Tumoral calcinosis. *Br. J. Radiol.*, 39: 518–23.

Chapter 10
Face and Neck

10.1   Unilateral Exophthalmos

Dysthyroid
This is the commonest cause, but most are diagnosed clinically.

Orbital Lesion
1. **Neoplasms** — child
   (a) Metastases — neuroblastoma, Ewing's, leukaemia, lymphoma.
   (b) Rhabdomyosarcoma — commonest primary orbital tumour in children. Metastasizes early to lung, bone, and brain.
   (c) Retinoblastoma — metastasizes late.
   (d) Optic nerve glioma.
2. **Neoplasms** — adult
   (a) Haemangioma — ± phleboliths.
   (b) Lymphoma.
   (c) Optic nerve glioma — age usually less than 35. Optic canal increased in size in 90%.
   (d) Orbital meningioma — age usually over 35. Optic canal increased in size in 10%.
   (e) Neurofibromatosis* — 'bare' orbit and widened superior orbital fissure.
   (f) Metastases — often show lytic bone changes.
   (g) Dermoid.
   (h) Lacrimal gland tumour.
3. **Vascular**
   (a) Arteriovenous malformation — ± phleboliths.
   (b) Haematoma — due to fracture/trauma.
4. **Granuloma (pseudotumour)** — obstruction of the cavernous sinus may occur (Tolosa–Hunt syndrome).

Intracranial Lesion
1. **Meningioma** — ± hyperostosis of the apex of the orbit, or lesser wing of sphenoid.
2. **Glioma**.
3. **Infraclinoid aneurysm**.
4. **Cavernous sinus thrombosis**.

Sinus/bone Lesion
1. **Fibrous dysplasia*** — leontiasis ossea of the antrum.
2. **Neoplasms**
   (a) Carcinoma of paranasal sinus.
   (b) Osteoma.
   (c) Dermoid — typical expansion of the superolateral part of the orbital roof.
3. **Mucocele** — extending inferiorly from the frontal sinus.
4. **Craniostenosis** (q.v.).

Further Reading
Price H.I. & Danziger A. (1979) The computerised tomographic findings in paediatric orbital tumours. *Clin. Radiol.*, 30: 435–40.

10.2   Enlarged Orbit
Exclude small contralateral orbit, e.g. enucleation as a child.

1. **Neurofibromatosis*** — ± 'bare' orbit due to elevation of the lesser wing of the sphenoid and associated dysplasia.
2. **Congenital glaucoma (buphthalmos)** — asymmetrical enlargement.
3. **Any space occupying lesion** — if present long enough. The enlargement in children occurs much faster. (See section 10.1.)

10.3   'Bare' Orbit

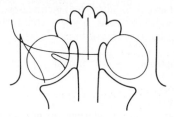

1. **Neurofibromatosis*** — dysplasia of the sphenoid.
2. **Metastasis** — bone destruction.
3. **Meningioma** — adjacent bone sclerosis.

Further Reading
Burrows E.H. (1963) Bone changes in orbital neurofibromatosis. *Br. J. Radiol.*, 36: 549–61.

10.4   Enlarged Optic Foramen

Diameter greater than 7 mm (normal range of 4.4–6 mm is reached by the age of four). However, the final arbiter is always comparison with the asymptomatic side. A difference in diameter of 1 mm is abnormal.

Concentric Enlargement
1. **Optic nerve glioma** — child/young adult. 25% associated with neurofibromatosis. Bone margins intact.
2. **Neurofibroma** — may occur without any associated glioma.
3. **Extension of retinoblastoma**.
4. **Vascular** — ophthalmic artery aneurysm, arterovenous malformation.
5. **Granuloma** — very rarely in sarcoid or pseudotumour.

Local Defect

ROOF

1. **Adjacent neoplasm** — meningioma, metastases, glioma.
2. **Raised intracranial pressure** (q.v.) — due to thinning of the floor of the anterior cranial fossa.

MEDIAL WALL

1. **Adjacent neoplasm** — carcinoma of the ethmoid/sphenoid.
2. **Sphenoid mucocele**.

INFEROLATERAL WALL

1. Same conditions as cause **enlargement of superior orbital fissure** (q.v.).

Further Reading

Lloyd G.A.S. (1975) *Radiology of the Orbit*, pp. 26–9. Philadelphia: Saunders.

10.5   Enlarged Superior Orbital Fissure

1. **Normal variant**.
2. **Neurofibromatosis***.
3. **Extension of intracranial lesion**
   (a) Meningioma — adjacent sclerosis.
   (b) Infraclinoid aneurysm — occurs in 75%. Usually accompanied by erosion of the inferior surface of the anterior clinoid.
   (c) Parasellar chordoma.
4. **Metastasis to wing of sphenoid**.
5. **Extension of orbital lesion (anterior clinoids not eroded)**
   (a) Arterovenous malformation.
   (b) Haemangioma.
   (c) Orbital meningioma.
   (d) Lymphoma.

10.6   Intraorbital Calcification

In the Globe
1. **Cataract.**
2. **Retinoblastoma** — young children. Very fine, stippled calcification. 30% are bilateral. ± proptosis. Siblings may also be affected.
3. **Old trauma/infection** — of the vitreous humour.

Outside the Globe
1. **Phleboliths**
   (a) Arteriovenous malformation — enlarged orbit and proptosis. ± prominent vascular markings. Can also occur in an arterovenous shunt (e.g. secondary to a traumatic carotico-cavernous fistula).
   (b) Haemangioma — only rarely have calcified phleboliths.
2. **Orbital meningioma** — 12% calcify (more common in extradural location). 20% show enlargement of the optic foramen. Sclerosis of the orbital apex may be present if extradural in location.
3. **Others** — rarely in neurofibroma, intraorbital dermoid and adenocarcinoma of the lacrimal gland.

10.7   Hyperostosis in the Orbit

1. **Meningioma.**
2. **Sclerotic metastases.**
3. **Fibrous dysplasia*** — bone expansion may cause some reduction in size of the orbit.
4. **Paget's disease*** — usually widespread changes in the calvarium.
5. **Chronic osteomyelitis** — adjacent to a chronically infected frontal sinus.
6. **Lacrimal gland malignancy.**
7. **Histiocytosis X*.**
8. **Radiotherapy.**

10.8   Small or Absent Sinuses

Congenital
1. **Congenital absence** — absence of the frontal sinuses occurs in 5% of the normal population.
2. **Cretinism***.
3. **Down's syndrome*** — 90% have absent frontal sinuses.
4. **Kartagener's syndrome** — dextrocardia, bronchiectasis and absent frontal sinuses.

Overgrowth of Bony Wall
1. **Paget's disease***.
2. **Fibrous dysplasia***.
3. **Haemolytic anaemia***.

10.9   Opaque Maxillary Antrum

Traumatic
1. **Fracture** — blood in the antrum.
2. **Overlying soft-tissue swelling** — gives apparent opacification of the antrum.
3. **Postoperative** — washout/Caldwell-Luc.
4. **Epistaxis**.
5. **Barotrauma**.

Inflammatory/Infective
1. **Infection**.
2. **Allergy**.
3. **Pyocele** — infected mucocele (rare in the antrum). Severe systemic symptoms.

Neoplastic
1. **Carcinoma** — ± bone destruction and extension of the soft-tissue mass.
2. **Lymphoma***

Others
1. **Fibrous dysplasia*** — ± bone expansion.
2. **Cysts** — dentigerous and mucous retention cysts may be large enough to fill the antrum.
3. **Wegener's granulomatosis**.
4. **Technical** — overtilted view.
5. **Anatomical** — thick skull vault, sloping antral wall.

10.10 Mass in the Maxillary Antrum

1. **Cysts**
   (a) Mucous retention cyst — complication of sinusitis. Maxillary antrum is a common site, and it often arises from the floor. Commoner than a polyp, but hard to differentiate between them.
   (b) Dentigerous cyst — expands upwards into the floor of the antrum. The involved tooth may be displaced into the antrum.
2. **Trauma** — due to 'tear-drop' of prolapsed muscle through the roof of the antrum in an orbital blow-out fracture.
3. **Neoplasms**
   (a) Polyp — complication of sinusitis.
   (b) Carcinoma — ± bone destruction and soft-tissue mass extending beyond the boundary of the antrum.
4. **Wegener's granulomatosis** — age usually 40–50. Early mucosal thickening progresses to a mass with bone destruction.

10.11 Loss of Lamina Dura of Teeth

Generalized
1. **Endocrine/metabolic**
   (a) Osteoporosis (q.v.).
   (b) Hyperparathyroidism*.
   (c) Cushing's syndrome*.
   (d) Osteomalacia (q.v.).
2. **Paget's disease***.
3. **Scleroderma*** — thickened periodontal membrane.

Localized
1. **Infection**.
2. **Neoplasms** — leukaemia, multiple myeloma, metastases, Burkitt's lymphoma, Histiocytosis X.

10.12   'Floating' Teeth

No obvious supporting bone for the teeth.

1. **Severe periodontal disease**.
2. **Histiocytosis X***.
3. **Hyperparathyroidism***.
4. **Metastes**.
5. **Multiple myeloma***.

10.13   Cystic Lesion in the Mandible

Dental
1. **Periodontal cyst** — periapical rounded lucency with a sclerotic margin. Due to chronic infection.
2. **Dentigerous cyst** — adjacent to the crown of an unerupted tooth (usually a wisdom tooth or canine). Multiple cysts occur in children with Gorlin's syndrome — multiple basal cell naevi which may become malignant. Autosomal dominant inheritance.

Non-dental
1. **Hyperparathyroidism** — common site for a brown tumour.
2. **Neoplasms**
   (a) Cystic adamantinoma — multilocular. Usually at the angle of the mandible.
   (b) Aneurysmal bone cyst*.
   (c) Giant cell tumour*.
   (d) Haemangioma.
   (e) Histiocytosis X*.
   (f) Metastases.
3. **Fibrous dysplasia*** — rare site.
4. **Bone cyst**.

10.14 Mass in the Nasopharynx

1. **Adenoids** — enlargement is normal between 1–7 years of age.
2. **Trauma** — fracture of the base of the skull or upper cervical spine with associated haematoma.
3. **Infection** — abscess may be confined above C2 by strong attachment of the prevertebral fascia. ± speckled gas in the mass.
4. **Neoplasms, benign**
   (a) Adolescent angiofibroma — very vascular. Young male — ± spontaneous regression after adolescence. Can cause pressure erosion of the sphenoid and opacification of the antra.
   (b) Antro-choanal polyp.
5. **Neoplasms, malignant**
   (a) Nasopharyngeal carcinoma.
   (b) Lymphoma*.
   (c) Rhabdomyosarcoma.
   (d) Plasmacytoma*.
   (e) Extension — carcinoma of the sphenoid/ethmoid, and chordoma.
6. **Encephalocele** — midline defect in the base of the skull.

10.15   Prevertebral Soft-tissue Mass in the Cervical Region

Child

N.B. Anterior buckling of the trachea, which may occur in expiration, flexion or oblique views, can simulate a prevertebral mass. An ear lobe may also mimic a prevertebral mass.

1. **Trauma/haematoma** — ± an associated fracture.
2. **Abscess** — ± gas lucencies within it.
3. **Neoplasms**
    (a) Neuroblastoma.
    (b) Teratoma.
    (c) Lymphoma*.
    (d) Cystic hygroma.

Adult

1. **Trauma**.
2. **Abscess**.
3. **Neoplasms**
    (a) Post-cricoid carcinoma.
    (b) Lymphoma*.
    (c) Chordoma.
4. **Pharyngeal pouch** — ± air/fluid level within it.
5. **Retropharyngeal goitre**.

See also section 10.14.

Chapter 11
Skull and Brain

11.1 Lucency in the Skull Vault, with No Surrounding Sclerosis — Adult

Neoplastic
1. **Multiple myeloma*** — involves cancellous and cortical bone, hence punched out appearance. It can affect the mandible (metastases rarely do) and paranasal sinuses. Lesions are cold on radioisotope bone-scan. The skull may be normal even with widespread lesions elsewhere.
2. **Metastases** — usually irregular and ill defined. Especially breast, kidney, thyroid.
3. **Haemangioma** — may have 'soap bubble' appearance, and can cause 'hair-on-end' appearance (q.v.).
4. **Neurofibroma** — may cause a lucent defect in the occipital bone (usually adjacent to the left lambdoid suture).
5. **Adjacent malignancy** — e.g. rodent ulcer, carcinoma of the ear.
6. **Paget's sarcoma**.

Traumatic
1. **Burr hole** — very well defined.

Idiopathic
1. **Osteoporosis circumscripta** — occurs in the active lytic phase of Paget's disease*. It starts in the lower part of the frontal and occipital regions (i.e. rare in the vertex) and can cross suture lines to involve large areas of the calvarium. Basilar invagination and loss of the lamina dura around the teeth may occur.
2. **Sarcoidosis*** — can occur without other bony lesions in the hands. Usually small and multiple with no sclerotic margin. Can affect inner and outer tables.

Metabolic
1. **Hyperparathyroidism*** — 'pepper pot skull'. Rarely severe
   enough to cause overt lytic lesions. The calvarium is
   affected in approximately 20% of primary hyperparathyroidism causing 'pepper pot' appearance. The mandible is a
   common site for 'brown' tumours and there may be loss of
   the lamina dura around the teeth. Basilar invagination may
   occur.

Infective
1. **Tuberculosis** — tuberculous osteomyelitis is much less
   common than tuberculous arthritis and the skull is a rare
   site (the spine being the most common). It can produce a
   punched out lytic lesion.
2. **Hydatid**.
3. **Syphilis** — 'moth-eaten' appearance.

11.2 Lucency in the Skull Vault, with no Surrounding Sclerosis — Child

Neoplastic
1. **Metastases** — especially neuroblastoma and leukaemia. ± wide sutures.
2. **Histiocytosis X*** — eosinophilic granuloma usually produces a solitary lesion which only causes local pain. It can have bevelled edges, due to differential destruction of the inner and outer tables, and can grow several centimetres in size in a few weeks. There is no sclerosis unless the lesion is healing.

    Hand–Schüller–Christian syndrome produces the 'geographical' skull, with associated systemic symptoms. Exophthalmos and diabetes insipidus accompany it in less than 10% of cases. Chronic otitis media, and loose teeth due to surrounding lucencies ('floating' teeth), commonly occur. 'Honeycomb lung' occurs in 10% of cases and worsens the prognosis.

Traumatic
1. **Leptomeningeal cyst** — if the dura is torn, the arachnoid membrane can prolapse, and the pulsations of the CSF can cause progressive widening and scalloping of the fracture line. The bone changes take several weeks to appear and may persist into adult life.
2. **Burr hole**.

N.B. Normal variants such as parietal foramina and venous lakes, apart from having characteristic configurations, will also be 'cold' on a radioisotope bone-scan.

11.3   Lucency in the Skull Vault, with Surrounding Sclerosis

*Fibrous Dysplasia**

Developmental
1. **Epidermoid** — scalloped appearance with thin sclerotic margins. It is intramedullary in origin and so can expand both inner and outer tables. Although any site is possible, it is commonly in the squamous portion of the occipital or temporal bones.
2. **Meningocele** — this is a mid-line defect and has a smooth sclerotic margin with an overlying soft-tissue mass. It usually occurs in the occipital bone, but may occur in the frontal, parietal or basal bones.

Neoplastic
1. **Haemangioma** — only rarely has a sclerotic margin. Radiating spicules of bone within it are a helpful discriminatory sign.
2. **Histiocytosis X*** — only has a sclerotic margin if it is in the healing phase.

Infective
1. **Chronic osteomyelitis** — sclerosis dominates, with only a few lytic areas.
2. **Frontal sinus mucocoele** — secondary to sinusitis.

Further Reading
Lane B. (1974) Erosions of the Skull. *Radiol. Clin. North Am.*, 12: 257–82.

11.4   Multiple Lucent Lesions in the Skull Vault

1. **Neoplasms**
    (a) Metastases.
    (b) Multiple myeloma*.
    (c) Histiocytosis X*.
2. **Osteomyelitis**.
    (a) Acute — multiple small ill-defined lucencies associated with frontal sinusitis mastoiditis, scalp wound or infected bone flap. There is no surrounding sclerosis or periosteal reaction.
    (b) Chronic — sclerosis becomes a feature.
3. **Avascular necrosis** — of bone flap is identical in appearance to acute osteomyelitis, but it is slower in progression and there is no clinical evidence of an infection.
4. **Radiotherapy** — can cause multiple small lucencies.
5. **Hyperparathyroidism*** — rarely produces overt lytic lesions.
6. **Sarcoidosis*** — can occur without bony lesions in hands. Usually small and multiple with no sclerotic reaction.

11.5 Generalized Increase in Density of the Skull Vault

1. **Paget's disease*** — multiple islands of dense bone. Later the differentiation between the inner and outer tables is lost and the skull vault is thickened (2–5 times normal). Basilar invagination may occur. The sinuses may be involved giving an appearance similar to leontiasis ossea. Loss of lamina dura may occur.
2. **Sclerotic metastases** (q.v.).
3. **Fibrous dysplasia*** — if the lesions are widespread throughout the skeleton, then the skull always has a lesion. However, if only the facial bones and base of skull are involved (leontiasis ossea), the rest of the skeleton is rarely affected. Younger age group than Paget's disease.
4. **Myelosclerosis** — there is endosteal thickening which causes narrowing of the diploë. The spleen is greatly enlarged.
5. **Renal osteodystrophy*** — osteosclerosis occurs in 25%. The skull and spine are commonly involved and can look similar to Paget's disease. ± vascular calcification.
6. **Fluorosis** — mottling of the tooth enamel is a pronounced feature. The calvarium is a rare site for changes to be seen, the axial skeleton being the most frequent. Calcification of muscle attachments.
7. **Acromegaly*** — enlarged frontal sinuses, prognathism, enlarged sella, thick vault.
8. **Phenytoin therapy**.
9. **Chronic haemolytic anaemias**.
10. **Congenital**
    (a) Osteopetrosis — 'bone in bone' appearance in the spine. The mandible is not affected. Flask-shaped femora.
    (b) Pyknodysostosis — particularly involves the skull base. Wormian bones. Wide sutures.
    (c) Pyle's disease — associated with metaphyseal splaying of the long bones.

°

11.6 Localized Increase in Density
of the Skull Vault

In Bone
1. **Neoplasms**
   (a) Sclerotic metastases (q.v.).
   (b) Osteoma — rare in vault. More common in frontal sinus (ivory osteoma).
   (c) Treated lytic metastases — especially breast primary.
   (d) Treated 'brown' tumour.
2. **Paget's disease***.
3. **Fibrous dysplasia***.
4. **Depressed fracture** — due to overlapping bone fragments.
5. **Benign hyperostosis** — commonly seen in post menopausal females (rare in men). Mainly involves the frontal region, and is characteristically bilateral and symmetrical. Thickening of inner table — 'choppy sea' appearance.

Adjacent to Bone
1. **Meningioma** — mainly involves the inner table, but if it breaks through the outer table it may cause a 'hair-on-end' appearance. About 15% show calcification in the tumour itself. There may be an abnormal increase in the vascular channels and also signs of raised intracranial pressure. The characteristic sites are parasagittal, olfactory groove, sphenoid ridge and tentorium.
2. **Calcified sebaceous cyst**.
3. **Old cephalhaematoma** — it is usually in the parietal region, and may be bilateral.
4. **Soft-tissue tumours** — e.g. neurofibroma, sebaceous cyst.
5. **Hair bunch**.

11.7 Increase in Density of the Skull Base

Localized
1. **Fibrous dysplasia***
2. **Meningioma**.
3. **Sclerotic metastases** (q.v.).
4. **Chronic suppurative otitis media**.

Generalized
1. **Paget's disease***.
2. **Fibrous dysplasia***.
3. **Other causes of generalized increase in bone density** (q.v.).

11.8   Destruction of Petrous Bone — Apex

1. **Acoustic neuroma** — eighth nerve. Increase in size of IAM (greater than 1 cm in diameter or more than 2 mm asymmetry between the sides). Erosion of the crista transversalis and apparent 'shortening' of the IAM may occur. Bilateral in neurofibromatosis.
2. **Congenital cholesteatoma** — lytic defect with no sclerosis. Petrous ridge may be elevated. Seventh nerve may be involved (this is rare in acoustic neuroma).
3. **Meningioma**.
4. **Metastases** — particularly breast, kidney and lung. Irregular lytic defect. Pain, bleeding and nerve palsy are common.
5. **Fifth nerve neuroma**.
6. **Nasopharyngeal carcinoma** — usually large area of destruction in the floor of the middle cranial fossa also.
7. **Chordoma**.
8. **Apical petrositis**.

Further Reading

Livingstone P.A. (1974) Differential diagnosis of radiolucent lesions of the temporal bone. *Radiol. Clin. North Am.*, 12: 571–83.

11.9 Destruction of Petrous Bone — Middle Ear

Adult

1. **Acquired cholesteatoma** — usually diagnosed by auroscopy. Bony destruction extending from the epitympanic recess, with clear cut but not sclerotic margins. Earliest sign is destruction of the spur (80%). Ossicles may be destroyed. The mastoid antrum is often sclerotic due to the associated chronic infection.

2. **Carcinoma of the middle ear** — 30% associated with chronic otitis media. Pain and bleeding are late. 12% show bony destruction (particularly of the articular fossa of the temporomandibular joint).

3. **Metastases**.

4. **Glomus jugulare** — the jugular foramen is enlarged and destroyed, with minimal or no sclerosis. Very vascular — can look like an aneurysm.

5. **Tuberculosis** — rare. Destruction with no sclerosis. May be no evidence of TB elsewhere.

Child

1. **Rhabdomyosarcoma** — commonest primary malignancy of ear in childhood. Pain is rare.

Further Reading

Phelps P.D. & Lloyd G.A.S. (1981) The radiology of carcinoma of the ear. *Br. J. Radiol.* 54: 103–9.

Phelps P.D. & Lloyd G.A.S. (1980) The radiology of cholesteatoma. *Clin. Radiol.* 31: 501–12.

Livingstone P.A. (1974) Differential diagnosis of radiolucent lesions of the temporal bone. *Radiol. Clin. North Am.*, 12: 571–83.

11.10　Basilar Invagination

McGregor's line (tip of hard palate to the base of the occiput). The tip of the odontiod peg is normally less than 0.5 cm above this line. If basilar invagination is severe obstructive hydrocephalus may occur.

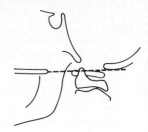

Primary Anomalies of the Occiput, Atlas and Axis

Generalized Bone Disease
1. **Rickets*/osteomalacia** (q.v.).
2. **Paget's disease*.**
3. **Fibrous dysplasia*.**

Delayed or Defective Cranial Ossification
1. **Osteogenesis imperfecta*.**
2. **Achondroplasia*.**
3. **Cleidocranial dysplasia*.**
4. **Cranial thinning in hydrocephalus.**

N.B.
1. **Platybasia** — does not always accompany basilar invagination, but occurs in similar circumstances. The index of this is the basal angle, normal < 140°. By itself it is symptomless, but if associated with basilar invagination, then obstructive hydrocephalus may occur.

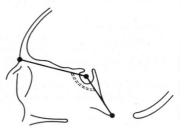

Basal angle

2. **Basilar invagination** — elevation of the floor of the posterior cranial fossa. This may be associated with anomalies of the cervical spine such as atlanto-occipital fusion or Klippel–Feil syndrome.

Further Reading
Dolan K.D. (1977) Cervicobasilar relationships. *Radiol. Clin. North Am.* 15: 155–66.

11.11   'Hair-on-end' Skull Vault

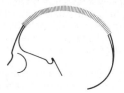

Haemolytic Anaemias
1. **Sickle-cell anaemia*** — occurs in 5%. Begins in the frontal region and can affect all the calvarium except that which is below the internal occipital protuberance, since there is no marrow in this area. The diploic space is widened due to marrow hyperplasia.
2. **Thalassaemia*** — marrow hyperplasia in thalassaemia major is more marked than in any other anaemia. May be severe enough to cause marrow hyperplasia of the facial bones, resulting in obliteration of the maxillary antra. (This does not occur in sickle-cell anaemia.)
3. **Others** — hereditary spherocytosis, elliptocytosis and pyruvate kinase deficiency.

Neoplastic
1. **Haemangioma**.
2. **Meningioma** — only rarely, when it breaks through the outer table.
3. **Neuroblastoma metastases** — may involve the sutures (particularly coronal suture) also, causing widening and irregularity. Orbital deposits causing proptosis are common.
4. **Osteosarcoma** — very rare.
5. **Plasmacytoma*** — spiculation may occur with the expansion of the diploë (usually parietal or occipital).

Others
1. **Cyanotic heart disease** — due to erythroid hyperplasia. Hypertrophic pulmonary osteoarthropathy may occur.
2. **Iron-deficiency anaemia** — severe childhood cases.

11.12   Craniostenosis

1. **Sutural fusion** — only a small segment of a suture may be
   fused, but this is sufficient to cause craniostenosis. The
   normal suture width is 1.5–10 mm at birth, falling to 2 mm at
   3 years. Fusion normally starts at about 22 years.
2. **Skull deformity** — the configuration will depend on which
   suture is fused:
   (a) Sagittal suture — scaphocephaly. A long, narrow 'boat-
       shaped' skull. This is the commonest type, is more
       common in boys and may be asymptomatic.
   (b) Coronal and lambdoid sutures — oxycephaly, turri-
       cephaly or acrocephaly. A high 'tower-' or 'turret-shaped'
       skull. This can cause proptosis, optic and VIII nerve
       lesions and signs of raised intracranial pressure.
   (c) Metopic suture — trigonocephaly. The frontal bone is
       pointed anteriorly due to in-utero fusion.
   (d) Generalized — microcephaly.
   (e) Asymmetrical — plagiocephaly.
3. **Raised intracranial pressure** (q.v.) — if the craniostenosis is
   long standing.

1. **Idiopathic**.
2. **Apert's syndrome (acrocephalosyndactyly)**
   (a) Acrocephaly.
   (b) Mental retardation (in some).
   (c) Fontanelles large and late in closure.
   (d) Shallow orbits, hypertelorism and maxillary hypo-
       plasia.
   (e) Osseous or cutaneous syndactyly.
   (f) Broad distal phalanx of thumb and great toe.
3. **Carpenter's syndrome (acrocephalopolysyndactyly)**
   (a) Acrocephaly.
   (b) Mental retardation.
   (c) Obesity.
   (d) Lateral displacement of the inner canthi.
   (e) Brachydactyly of the hands, with clinodactyly and
       partial syndactyly.
   (f) Polydactyly of the feet, with partial syndactyly.

4. **Crouzon's syndrome (craniofacial dysostosis)**
   (a) Craniostenosis of the coronal, lambdoid and sagittal sutures.
   (b) Proptosis due to shallow orbits.
   (c) Frontal bossing.
   (d) Maxillary hypoplasia.
5. **Hypophosphatasia (infantile form)*** — sutures are initially widened.

11.13 Wormian Bones

1. **Osteogenesis imperfecta*** — autosomal dominant (with variable penetrance) 'tam-o'-shanter' skull deformity.
2. **Cleidocranial dysplasia*** — autosomal dominant. Brachycephaly with open sutures and anterior fontanelle. The teeth are always poorly formed/delayed and multiple supernumerary teeth may be present. Small facial bones.
3. **Pyknodysostosis** — autosomal recessive. Short-limbed dwarf, with some features of osteopetrosis and cleidocranial dysplasia.
4. **Hypophosphatasia*** — autosomal recessive. Low alkaline phosphatase, and excessive phosphoethanolamine in the urine. Premature fusion of the sutures.
5. **Cretinism*** — delayed, fragmented epiphyses. There is usually a hypoplastic 'bullet-shaped' vertebra at L1 or L2 level.
6. **Primary acro-osteolysis** — brachycephaly, open sutures, severe basilar invagination.
7. **Down's syndrome***.

11.14   Raised Intracranial Pressure

Child

1. **Suture diastasis** — occurs easily up to the age of 8 years and may take only a few days to appear. Particularly noticeable in coronal and sagittal sutures. (Maximum normal width: 1 cm at birth, 2 mm at 3 years.) If chronic, excess interdigitations may be seen.
2. **Increased head size**.
3. **Craniolacunia** — oval/finger-shaped pits on inner table, with bony ridges between. Seen in the neonate and gradually fade by 6 months. Associated with myelomeningocoele, encephalocoele, aqueduct stenosis and Arnold–Chiari malformation.
4. **Erosion of the dorsum sellae** — late sign (takes several weeks to develop). Only seen in 30%. If no associated, suture diastasis, then look for parasellar pathology.
5. **Increased convolutional markings** — unreliable. Normal variant age 4–10 years.

Adult

1. **Erosion of the dorsum sellae** — occurs earliest at the base of the dorsum sellae.
2. **Pineal displacement** — if the raised intracranial pressure is due to a space occupying lesion.
3. **Calcification** — may occur in space occupying lesion.

N.B. If symptoms have been present for longer than 5 weeks, then 30% have signs on SXR. Headache and papilloedema may be absent even in the presence of signs on the SXR.

1. **Space-occupying lesion**
   (a) Tumour.
   (b) Abscess.
   (c) Haematoma — intracerebral, extra/subdural.
2. **Obstructive hydrocephalus**
   (a) Communicating — e.g. post-meningitis/subarachnoid haemorrhage, superior sagittal sinus thrombosis.
   (b) Non-communicating — e.g. congenital stenosis, SOL causing obstruction to ventricular pathway.
3. **Craniostenosis**.
4. **Cerebral oedema**.
5. **Toxic** — e.g. lead.

11.15 Large Heads and Ventricles in Infants

Large Head
1. **Large ventricles**
   (a) Hydrocephalus — most commonly due to aqueduct stenosis, Arnold–Chiari malformation or Dandy–Walker cyst.
2. **Normal ventricles**
   (a) Abnormal vault shape.
   (b) Cerebral oedema.
   (c) Intracranial space-occupying lesion.
   (d) Megalencephaly.

Large Ventricles
1. **Large head**
   (a) Hydrocephalus.
2. **Normal-sized head**
   (a) Cerebral atrophy — most commonly due to intrauterine infection, natal/postnatal anoxia or arterial/venous occlusions.

Further Reading
Harwood-Nash D.C. & Fitz C.R. (1975) Large heads and ventricles in infants. *Radiol. Clin. North Am.* 13: 199–224.

11.16 Wide Sutures

1. At Birth — suture width greater than 1 cm.
2. At 3 years — suture width greater than 2 mm.

Raised Intracranial Pressure (q.v.)
Suture diastasis only if onset before 10 years age.

1. **Space-occupying lesion**.
2. **Hydrocephalus**.

Infiltration of the Sutures
1. **Neuroblastoma** — ± lucencies in skull vault and 'sunray' spiculation (a reaction to subpericranial deposits).
2. **Leukaemia** ⎫ — in children.
3. **Lymphoma*** ⎭

Defective Ossification

1. **Rickets***.
2. **Renal osteodystrophy***.
3. **Cleidocranial dysplasia***.
4. **Osteogenesis imperfecta***.
5. **Hypophosphatasia*** — premature fusion of sutures later, resulting in craniostenosis.

11.17   Pneumocephalus

1. **Trauma** — fracture of the ethmoid or frontal sinuses is commonest. Fluid levels in sinus. Dural tear permits CSF rhinorrea (positive for glucose).
2. **Iatrogenic** — postoperative/air encephalogram.
3. **Abscess**.
4. **Osteoma** — if erodes cribriform plate.
5. **Nasopharyngeal/ethmoid carcinoma**.

11.18   Small Pituitary Fossa

1. **Normal variant**.
2. **Dystrophia myotonica** — hereditary. Usually starts in early adult life. Cataracts, frontal baldness, testicular atrophy, thick skull and large frontal sinus.
3. **Radiotherapy as child**.
4. **Hypopituitarism**.

11.19   Expanded Pituitary Fossa

1. **Size** — normal range is : height 6.5–11 mm
                                        length 9–16 mm
                                        breadth 9–19 mm
1. **Double floor** — can be a normal variant (asymmetrical development), but a tumour should be suspected.
3. **Elevation/destruction of clinoid processes**.
4. **Loss of lamina dura**.

1. **Para/intrasellar mass**.
   (a) Pituitary adenoma
       (i) Chromophobe (non-functioning); commonest cause of expansion and commonest adenoma to produce suprasellar extension. 10% do not expand the sella.
       (ii) eosinophilic (acromegaly); only slight expansion.
       (iii) basophilic (Cushing's syndrome); virtually never expands.
   (b) Craniopharyngioma — 50% cause expansion — usually slight.
   (c) Prolactinoma — typically a blister on the antero-inferior wall. SXR abnormal in 20%. Tomography detects abnormality in 50%. CT useful for detecting suprasellar extension.
       N.B. Other causes of hyperprolactinaemia are:
       (i) Physiological — pregnancy.
       (ii) Drugs — phenothiazines, tricyclics, methyldopa, metoclopramide and oral contraceptives.
       (iii) Hypothalamic and stalk lesions — encephalitis, tumours, trauma and histiocytosis X.
       (iv) Severe hypothyroidism.
       (v) Renal failure.
   (d) Meningioma — usually produces sclerosis, but may cause erosion and expansion of the sella.
   (e) Aneurysm — well-defined pressure resorption of bone ± curvilinear calcification.
2. **Raised intracranial pressure** (q.v.) — due to dilated third ventricle.

3. **Empty sella**
   (a) Primary — defect in diaphragma sellae allows pulsating CSF to expand the sella. Typically obese with hypertension. Headache common. Visual and endocrine defects uncommon. Associated with benign intracranial hypertension. SXR abnormal in 85% — symmetrical expansion with no erosion.
   (b) Secondary — pituitary tumour or treatment of a pituitary lesion may distort the diaphragma sellae.
4. **Nelson's syndrome** — post adrenalectomy for Cushing's syndrome.

Further Reading

Doyle F.H. (1979) Radiology of the pituitary fossa. In: Lodge T. & Steiner R.E. (eds) *Recet Advances in Radiology*, Vol. 6, pp. 121–43. Edinburgh, Churchill Livingstone.
Sage M.R., Chan E.S.H. & Reilly P.L. (1980) The clinical and radiological features of the empty sella syndrome. *Clin. Radiol.*, 31: 513–19.
Teasdale E., Macpherson P. & Teasdale G. (1981) The reliability of radiology in detecting prolactin-secreting pituitary microadenomas. *Brit. J. Radiol.*, 54: 566–71.

11.20   Erosion and Osteoporosis of the Sella, with no Expansion

1. **Erosion** — the earliest sign is interruption of the lamina dura at the base of the dorsum sellae. The line of the lamina dura should normally be complete, even in the elderly, and any defect is significant.
2. **Osteoporosis** (q.v.) — the cortex may become blurred.

Raised Intracranial Pressure (q.v.) — commonest cause of erosion. (In children, suture diastasis is a more prominent sign.) 30% show this if raised ICP has been present more than 5–6 weeks. In 20% of those with X-ray changes papilloedema is not present.

Parasellar Masses
1. **Craniopharyngioma**.
2. **Meningioma**.
3. **Pituitary adenoma**.
4. **Aneurysm**.
5. **Chordoma**.
6. **Metastases** — kidney, bronchus, breast, prostate, malignant melanoma.
7. **Local invasion** — (e.g. carcinoma of the sphenoid or nasopharynx).

Generalized Decrease in Bone Density
1. **Osteoporosis** (q.v.).
2. **Osteomalacia** (q.v.).
3. **Hyperparathyroidism***.

Malignant Hypertension

11.21   J-shaped Sella

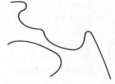

Flattened tuberculum sellae with a
prominent sulcus chiasmaticus. Rare
in adults.

1. **Normal variant** — 5% of normal children.
2. **Optic chiasm glioma** — if the chiasmatic sulcus is markedly depressed (W- or omega-shaped sella), the tumour may be bilateral.
3. **Chronic hydrocephalus** — due to downward pressure of an enlarged third ventricle.
4. **Mucopolysaccharidoses**.
5. **Achondroplasia***.
6. **Neurofibromatosis*** — sphenoid dysplasia.

11.22   Unifocal Intracranial Calcification

Physiological — pineal, choroid plexus, etc.

Neoplastic
1. **Glioma** — overall 5–10% calcify, especially if slow growing. About 20% of astrocytomas and 50% of oligodendro-gliomas calcify (the latter being typically serpiginous in form), but astrocytomas are much more common.
2. **Meningioma** — 15% calcify (characteristically homogeneous and rounded) in psammoma bodies. Hyperostosis and an increase in the vascular channels may be seen.
3. **Metastases** — may occasionally calcify, particularly from colon, breast and osteosarcoma.
4. **Craniopharyngioma** — 90% calcify in children and 40% in adults. Two types — solid (walnut sized) and cystic (may be very large). The sella is abnormal (expanded or eroded) in 50%.
5. **Chordoma** — 50% show dense calcification adjacent to the clivus. 50% erode the clivus and reactive bone sclerosis may occur at the margins. 30% have a nasopharyngeal mass. Skeletal metastases may occur.
6. **Others**
   (a) Pituitary adenoma (chromophobe) — 1–6% calcify.
   (b) Pinealoma — suspect if pineal calcification is greater than 1 cm in diameter or occurs below the age of ten.
   (c) Lipoma — characteristically two curvilinear bands of calcification, one on each side of the corpus callosum.
   (d) Hamartoma — usually in temporal lobe.
   (e) Teratoma — 50% occur in the pineal region and usually present in the first decade of life.
   (f) Dermoid — majority in the midline of the posterior cranial fossa (cerebellar vermis, fourth ventricle, and base of skull). Usually presents in adolescence.
   (g) Epidermoid — majority not in the midline. Cerebello-pontine angle is the commonest site. These inclusions can also occur in the skull vault.
   (h) Choroid plexus papilloma — the commonest site is the fourth ventricle in children, and the temporal horn of the lateral ventricle in adults.

Vascular
1. **Atherosclerosis** — usually carotid siphon.
2. **Aneurysm** — 1% calcify. (Most patients present with subarachnoid haemorrhage and these aneurysms virtually never show calcification.) However, 'giant' aneurysms greater than 2.5 cm in diameter show curvilinear calcification in 50% of cases and are large enough to cause erosion of the sella in 20%.
3. **Arteriovenous malformations** — 15% calcify. Vascular grooves may be prominent.
4. **Chronic subdural haematoma** — 1–5% calcify. 15% bilateral. Usually parietal region.
5. **Old infarct**.
6. **Sturge–Weber syndrome** — capillary and venous angiomas associated with ipsilateral cutaneous 'port wine' naevus. The calcification is gyriform and occurs in the occipital/parietal region. The hemicranium is smaller on the affected side. Association with coarctation of the aorta.

Infective
1. **Abscess** — calcification occurs late. Usually frontal/temporal regions.
2. **Tuberculoma** — 1–5% calcify. Usually multiple but can be solitary.
3. **Tuberculous meningitis** — 50% of those children who recover show calcification which is usually in the thickened basal meninges. It takes 15 months – 3 years to develop. Obstructive hydrocephalus is common.

Extracerebral (i.e. mimics intracranial calcification)
1. **Calcified sebaceous cyst**.
2. **Osteoma of the calvarium**.
3. **Foreign body**.

11.23 Multifocal Intracranial Calcification

Infective

1. **Toxoplasmosis** — transplacental infection of the fetus. 80% show nodular calcification in infancy (cortical, basal ganglia, periventricular). Microcephaly, dilated ventricles and bilateral choroidoretinitis are usually present.
2. **Cytomegalovirus/rubella** — may be indistinguishable from toxoplasmosis, but tends to be more periventricular in distribution.
3. **Cysticercosis** — calcification occurs in the dead cysts of *Taenia solium*, and takes 1–10 years to develop. It is always supratentorial and is about 0.5 cm in size. Only 5% of infections produce cysts in the brain.
4. **Hydatid** — only 2% of infections produce cysts in the brain and these rarely calcify.
5. **Others** — tuberculomata, histoplasmosis, coccidiomycosis, cryptococcosis, torulosis, paragonimiasis.

Metabolic

1. **Hypo-, pseudohypo- and pseudopseudohypoparathyroid-ism*** — characteristically basal ganglia.
2. **Chronic renal failure**.
3. **Excess vitamin D**.
4. **Toxic** — lead, carbon monoxide.

Tuberous Sclerosis*

Scattered nodular calcification (mm's – 1 cm in size). Cortical and periventricular. The nodules may bulge into the ventricle. Calcification not visible until 2 years old. 15% develop glioma (characteristically at the foramen of Munro) in adolescence. Multiple hamartomas occur in other organs, particularly kidney. Periosteal thickening may be seen in the phalanges.

11.24 Parasellar Calcification

Neoplastic
1. **Craniopharyngioma**.
2. **Meningioma**.
3. **Pituitary adenoma** (chromophobe).
4. **Chordoma**.
5. **Optic chiasm glioma**.
6. **Cholesteatoma**.

Vascular
1. **Aneurysm** — circle of Willis or basilar artery.
2. **Atheroma** — carotid siphon.

Infective
1. **Tuberculous meningitis** — calcification in the basal meninges.

11.25 Basal Ganglia Calcification

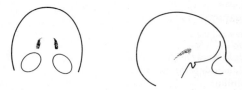

Idiopathic
Accounts for over 50% of cases and can be familial.

Metabolic
1. **Hypoparathyroidism*** — commonest pathological cause. Low serum calcium.
2. **Pseudohypoparathyroidism*** — short 4th and 5th metacarpals. End organ unresponsiveness to parathormone.
3. **Pseudopseudohypoparathyroidism***.
4. **Hyperparathyroidism***.

Infective
1. **Congenital cytomegalovirus.**
2. **Congenital toxoplasmosis.**

Poisoning
1. **Lead.**
2. **Carbon monoxide.**

Others
1. **Tuberous sclerosis*.**
2. **Fahr's disease** — presents in childhood with choreoathe-toid movements and progressive mental deterioration.
3. **Cockayne's syndrome** — microcephaly and truncal dwarf-ism. Progeria. Also has cortical calcification.

11.26   Curvilinear Calcification

Vascular
1. **Aneurysm.**
2. **Atheroma.**
3. **Angioma.**
4. **Haematoma.**

Neoplastic
1. **Cystic glioma** (astrocytoma).
2. **Cystic craniopharyngioma.**
3. **Teratoma.**
4. **Lipoma of corpus callosum.**

11.27   Posterior Cranial Fossa Neoplasms

Account for 30% of intrinsic brain tumours and 70% of childhood brain tumours.

CHILD

Midline
1. **Medulloblastoma** — vermis. Rapid growth and can seed along the spine. Radiosensitive.
2. **Choroid plexus papilloma** — fourth ventricle.

Lateral
1. **Astrocytoma** — cerebellar hemisphere and pons. Slow growth. Commonest posterior fossa tumour in childhood.

ADULT

Midline
1. **Glioma** — brain stem.
2. **Ependymoma** — lining of fourth ventricle.
3. **Choroid plexus papilloma** — fourth ventricle.
4. **Dermoid**.
5. **Chordoma**.

Lateral
1. **Metastases**.
2. **Cerebello–pontine angle tumours**
   (a) Acoustic neuroma.
   (b) Meningioma.
   (c) Cholesteatoma.
3. **Haemangioblastoma** — occasionally multiple, and associated with other angiomas (Hippel–Lindau syndrome).

11.28   CT Attenuation of Cerebral Masses
(relative to normal brain)

Hyperdense
1. **Neoplasms**
   - (a) Meningioma 95%.
   - (b) Microglioma (primary lymphoma).
   - (c) Metastases 30%.
   - (d) Glioma 10% (most glioblastomas show mixed attenuation).
   - (e) Ependymoma.
   - (f) Papilloma.
   - (g) Medulloblastoma 80%.
   - (h) Pituitary adenoma 25%.
   - (i) Craniopharyngioma (if solid).
   - (j) Acoustic neuroma 5%.
2. **Haematoma** — if ≤ 2 weeks old.
3. **Giant aneurysm**.
4. **Colloid cyst** — 50%.

Isodense
1. **Neoplasms**
   - (a) Acoustic neuroma 95%.
   - (b) Pituitary adenoma 65%.
   - (c) Glioma 10%.
   - (d) Metastases 10%.
   - (e) Chordoma.
   - (f) Pinealoma.
2. **Haematoma** — if 2–4 weeks old.
3. **Tuberculoma**.
4. **Colloid cyst** — 50%.

Hypodense
1. **Tumours**
   - (a) Craniopharyngioma.
   - (b) Glioma (95% of astrocytomas).
   - (c) Metastases 30%.
   - (d) Prolactinoma.
   - (e) Haemangioblastoma.
   - (f) Lipoma.
   - (g) Epidermoid.
   - (h) Dermoid.

2. **Haematoma** — ± if > 4 weeks old.
3. **Abscess** — pyogenic.
4. **Tuberculoma**.
5. **Cyst**
   (a) Arachnoid.
   (b) Porencephalic.
   (c) Hydatid.

11.29   CT Appearances of Cerebral Masses

A.

Tumours	Attenuation (μ)	Surrounding oedema	Contrast enhancement
Glioma	Increased or decreased (if cystic/necrotic)	Yes	95% if high grade; relatively infrequent in low grade; often *irregular ring*, but may be homogeneous or patchy
Metastases	Increased or decreased; often multifocal	Yes, extensive	Marked; may be *irregular ring*, homogeneous or patchy
Meningioma	Increased; multifocal in 5%	Minimal, perifocal (moderate in 20%)	Marked, homogeneous
Microglioma (i.e. primary lymphoma)	Increased (occasionally decreased, infiltrating); multifocal 50%	Yes	Marked, homogeneous
Pituitary adenoma	Isodense 65%; increased 25%	No	Marked, homogeneous
Prolactinoma	Hypodense	No	No
Craniopharyngioma	Decreased if cystic; increased if solid	No	± moderate homogeneous (solid), or *ring* (cystic)
Pinealoma	Isodense	No	Marked, homogeneous
Acoustic neuroma	Isodense 95%; increased 5%	No	Marked, homogeneous
Epidermoid (cholesteatoma)	Decreased	No	No
Medulloblastoma	Increased	Minimal, perifocal	Moderate, homogeneous
Haemangioblastoma	Decreased	Minimal	Moderate, homogeneous

Dermoid	Decreased	No	No
Chordoma	Isodense, poorly defined	No	Variable
Lipoma	Decreased	No	No
Papilloma	Increased	No	Marked, homogeneous
Ependymoma	Increased	May occur	± patchy
Glomus jugulare	Isodense	No	Moderate

B.

Infections	*Attenuation (µ)*	*Surrounding oedema*	*Contrast enhancement*
Pyogenic abscess	Decreased	Yes	*Regular ring* (thin walled)
Tuberculoma	Decreased or isodense; often multifocal	Yes	*Regular or irregular ring*; ± central ('target') enhancement characteristic
Hydatid	Decreased	No	No

C.

Vascular	*Attenuation (µ)*	*Surrounding oedema*	*Contrast enhancement*
Giant aneurysm	Increased	No	*Ring* or homogeneous
Arteriovenous malformation	± patchy increased	± patchy low attenuation due to surrounding infarcts	± marked, sinuous
Haematoma	Increased if fresh (isodense at 2 weeks; ± decreased at 4 weeks)	No	No (some peripheral enhancement may occur during the resorption phase)

D.

Cysts	Attenuation (µ)	Surrounding oedema	Contrast enhancement
Colloid	Increased 50%; isodense 50%	No	No
Arachnoid	Decreased (CSF)	No	No
Porencephalic	Decreased (CSF)	No	No

Further Reading

Lange S., Grumme T. & Meese W. (1980) *Computerized Tomography of the Brain.* Berlin: Schering A.G. Medico-scientific book series.

Bibliography

duBoulay G.H. (1980) *Principles of X-Ray Diagnosis of the Skull*, 2nd edn. London: Butterworths.

Chase N.E. & Kricheff I.I. (eds) (1974) The skull and brain. *Radiol. Clin. North Am.*, 12(2).

Felson B. (ed.) (1974) The normal skull and its variations. *Semin. Roentgenol.*, 9(2).

Leeds N.E. (ed.) (1982) Neuroradiology. *Radiol. Clin. North Am.*, 20(1).

Sutton D. (ed.) (1980) *Textbook of Radiology and Imaging*, 3rd edn., chaps 56–8, 63–4. Edinburgh: Churchill Livingstone.

PART 2

Achondroplasia

A primary defect of enchondral bone formation. Autosomal dominant (but 80% are spontaneous mutations).

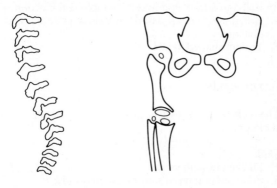

Skull
1. Large skull, Small base. Small sella. Steep clivus. Small funnel-shaped foramen magnum.
2. Hydrocephalus — of variable severity (± obstruction).

Thorax
1. Thick, stubby sternum.
2. Short ribs with deep concavities to the anterior ends.

Axial Skeleton
1. Decreasing interpedicular distance caudally in the lumbar spine.
2. Short pedicles with a narrow sagittal diameter of the lumbar spinal canal.
3. Disc height/body height ratio is 1.0 (normal 0.3).
4. Posterior scalloping.
5. Anterior vertebral body beak at T12/L1/L2.

Pelvis
1. Square iliac wings.
2. 'Champagne-glass' pelvic cavity.
3. Short, narrow sacrosciatic notch.
4. Horizontal sacrum articulating low on the ilia.

Appendicular Skeleton
1. Rhizomelic micromelia with bowing of long bones.
2. Widened metaphyses.
3. Ball-and-socket epiphyseal/metaphyseal junction.
4. Broad and short proximal and short proximal and middle phalanges.
5. Trident shaped hands.

Acromegaly

The effect of excessive growth hormone on the mature skeleton.

Skull
1. Thickened skull vault.
2. Enlarged paranasal sinuses and mastoids.
3. Enlarged pituitary fossa because of the eosinophilic adenoma.
4. Prognathism (increased angle of mandible).

Thorax and Spine
1. Increased sagittal diameter of the chest with a kyphosis.
2. Vertebral bodies show an increase in the AP and transverse dimensions with posterior scalloping.

Appendicular Skeleton
1. Increased width of bones but unaltered cortical thickness.
2. Tufting of the terminal phalanges.
3. Prominent muscle attachments.
4. Widened joint spaces—especially the metacarpo-pha-langeal joints—because of cartilage hypertrophy.
5. Premature osteoarthritis.
6. Increased heel pad thickness (> 21.5 mm in female; > 23 mm in male).
7. Generalized osteoporosis.

Alkaptonuria

The absence of homogentisic acid oxidase leads to the accumulation of homogentisic acid and its excretion in sweat and urine. The majority of cases are inherited as an autosomal recessive trait.

Axial Skeleton
1. Osteoporosis.
2. Intervertebral disc calcification — predominantly in the lumbar spine.
3. Disc space narrowing with vacuum phenomenon.
4. Marginal osteophytes and end-plate sclerosis.
5. Symphysis pubis — joint-space narrowing, chondrocalcinosis, eburnation and, rarely, bony ankylosis.

Appendicular Skeleton
1. Large joints show joint-space narrowing, bony sclerosis, articular collapse and fragmentation and intra-articular loose bodies.
2. Calcification of bursae and tendons.

Extraskeletal
Ochronotic deposition in other organs may have the following results

1. Cardiovascular system — atherosclerosis, infarction and murmurs.
2. Genitourinary system — prostatic enlargement with calculi.
3. Upper respiratory tract — hoarseness and dyspnoea.
4. Gastrointestinal tract — dysphagia.

Aneurysmal Bone Cyst

1. Age — 10–30 years (75% occur before epiphyseal closure).
2. Sites — ends of long bones, especially in the lower limbs. Also flat bones and vertebral appendages.
3. Appearances
   (a) Arises in unfused metaphysis or in metaphysis and epiphysis after fusion.
   (b) Well-defined lucency with thin but intact cortex.
   (c) Marked expansion (ballooning).
   (d) Thin internal strands of bone.
   (e) ± new bone in the angle between original cortex and the expanded part.

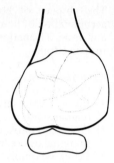

Ankylosing Spondylitis

A mesenchymal disease mainly manifest as an inflammatory arthritis affecting synovial and cartilaginous joints and as an enthesopathy.

Axial Skeleton
1. Involved initially in 70–80%. Initial changes in the sacroiliac joints followed by the thoracolumbar and lumbosacral regions. The entire spine may be involved eventually.
2. The radiological changes in the sacroiliac joints (see section 3.12) are present at the time of the earliest spinal changes.

3. Disco-vertebral junction
   (a) Osteitis — resulting in the squaring of vertebral bodies.
   (b) Syndesmophytes — eventually leading to the 'bamboo spine' (see section 2.13).
   (c) Disc calcification.
   (d) Erosions and destruction — which can be central, peripheral or extensive (pseudarthrosis).
   (e) Osteoporosis — with long-standing disease.
   (f) Kyphosis.
4. Apophyseal joints ⎫ haziness, erosions, subchondral
5. Costotransverse joints ⎬ sclerosis and eventually
6. Costovertebral joints ⎭ ankylosis.
7. Posterior ligament calcification and ossification.

Appendicular Skeleton
1. Involved initially in 10–20% but eventually in 50% of cases. Mild and transient. Asymmetrical involvement of few joints, most frequently hips and shoulders.
2. Similar changes to rheumatoid arthritis, but synovitis is more discrete and less severe. Subchondral bone sclerosis and chondral ossification lead to bony ankylosis. (In adult rheumatoid arthritis, bony ankylosis only occurs in the carpus and tarsus.)
3. No periarticular osteoporosis.

Extraskeletal
1. Iritis in 20% — more frequent with a peripheral arthropathy.
2. Pulmonary upper lobe fibrosis and cavitation (1%).
3. Heart disease — aortic incompetence, conduction defects and pericarditis.
4. Amyloidosis.
5. Inflammatory bowel disease.

Asbestosis

Lung and/or pleural disease due to the inhalation of asbestos fibres. Disease is more common with crocidolite (blue asbestos) than chrysotile (white asbestos). Pleural disease alone 50%; pleura and lung parenchyma 40%; lung parenchyma alone 10%.

Pleura
1. Plaques or pleural thickening. Most frequent in the lower half of the thorax and tend to follow rib contours. Parietal pleura is affected. Do not occur with less than 20 years exposure.
2. Calcified plaques (in 25%) — probably related to the type of fibre. Usually diaphragmatic.
3. Effusions (in 20%) — frequently recurrent, usually bilateral and often associated with chest pain. Usually associated with pulmonary involvement.

Lung Parenchyma
1. Small nodular and/or reticular opacities which progress through three stages
   (a) Fine reticulation in the lower zones → ground glass appearance.
   (b) More prominent interstitial reticulation in the lower zones.
   (c) Reticular shadowing in the mid and upper zones with obscured heart and diaphragmatic outlines.
2. Large opacities (1 cm or greater), associated with widespread interstitial fibrosis.

Complications
1. Carcinoma of the bronchus — 6–10× increased incidence in smokers with asbestosis and accounts for 35% of deaths.
2. Mesothelioma — 80% of all mesotheliomas are associated with asbestosis. Accounts for 10% of deaths.
3. Peritoneal mesothelioma.
4. Gastrointestinal carcinomas.
5. Laryngeal carcinoma.

Calcium Pyrophosphate Dihydrate Deposition Disease

1. Three manifestations which occur singly or in combination
   (a) Crystal-induced acute synovitis (pseudogout).
   (b) Cartilage calcification (chondrocalcinosis).
   (c) Structural joint abnormalities (pyrophosphate arthropathy).
2. Associated conditions are hyperparathyroidism and haemochromatosis (definite) and gout, Wilson's disease and alkaptonuria (less definite).
3. Chondrocalcinosis involves
   (a) Fibrocartilage — especially menisci of the knee, triangular cartilage of the wrist, symphysis pubis and annulus fibrosus of the intervertebral disc.
   (b) Hyaline cartilage — especially the wrist, knee, elbow and hip.
4. Synovial membrane, joint capsule, tendon and ligament calcification.
5. Pyrophosphate arthropathy is most common in the knee, wrist, metacarpophalangeal joint and acromioclavicular joint. It has similar appearances to osteoarthritis but with several differences
   (a) Unusual articular distribution — the wrist, elbow and shoulder are uncommon sites for osteoarthritis.
   (b) Unusual intra-articular distribution, e.g. the patello-femoral compartment of the knee and the radiocarpal compartment of the wrist.
   (c) Numerous, prominent subchondral cysts.
   (d) Marked subchondral collapse and fragmentation with multiple loose bodies simulating a neuropathic joint.
   (e) Variable osteophyte formation.

Chondroblastoma

1. Age — 5–20 years.
2. Sites — upper humerus, lower femur, upper tibia and greater tuberosity (50% occur in the lower limb).
3. Appearances
   (a) Arises in the epiphysis prior to fusion and may expand to involve the metaphysis.
   (b) Well-defined lucency with a thin sclerotic rim.
   (c) Internal calcification.

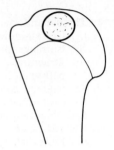

Chondromyxoid Fibroma

1. Age — 10–30 years.
2. Sites — upper end of tibia (50%); also femur and ribs.
3. Appearances
   (a) Metaphyseal ± extension into epiphysis, but never only in the epiphysis.
   (b) Round or oval, well-defined lucency with a sclerotic rim.
   (c) Eccentric expansion.
   (d) Internal calcification is uncommon.

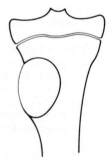

Chondrosarcoma

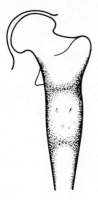

Central

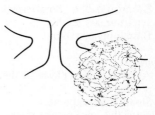

Central

1. Age — 30–60 years.
2. Sites — femur and humerus.
3. Appearances
   (a) Metaphyseal or diaphyseal.
   (b) Lucent, expansile lesion with a sclerotic margin.
   (c) Endosteal cortical thickening or thinning.
   (d) ± cortical destruction and a soft-tissue mass.
   (e) Amorphous or punctate internal calcification.

Peripheral

1. Age — 30–60 years.
2. Sites — pelvic and shoulder girdle, upper femur and humerus.
3. Appearances
   (a) Soft-tissue mass, often arising from the cartilage tip of an osteochondroma.
   (b) Multiple calcific densities.
   (c) Ill-defined margins.
   (d) In the later stages, destruction of underlying bone.

Cleidocranial Dysplasia

Autosomal dominant. One-third are new mutations.

Skull
1. Brachycephaly. Wormian bones. Frontal and parietal bossing.
2. Wide sutures and fontanelles with delayed closure.
3. Broad mandible. Small facial bones. Delayed eruption and supernumary teeth.
4. Basilar invagination.

Thorax
1. Aplasia or hypoplasia of the clavicles, usually the lateral portion.
2. Small, high scapulae.
3. Neonatal respiratory distress because of thoracic cage deformity.

Pelvis
1. Absent or delayed ossification of the pubic bones, producing apparent widening of the symphysis pubis.

Appendicular Skeleton
1. Short or absent fibulae.
2. Coxa vara or coxa valga.
3. Congenital pseudarthrosis of the femur.
4. Hand
   (a) Long 2nd and 5th metacarpals; short 2nd and 5th middle phalanges.
   (b) Cone-shaped epiphyses.
   (c) Acro-osteolysis.
   (d) Supernumerary ossification centres.

Coal Miner's Pneumoconiosis

The effect of the inhalation of coal dust in coal workers.

Simple
1. Small round opacities, 1–5 mm in size. Widespread throughout the lungs but sparing the extreme bases and apices.
2. Less well defined than silicosis.
3. Generally less dense than silicosis, but calcification occurs in at least a few of the nodules in 10% of older coal workers.
4. 'Eggshell' calcification of lymph nodes in 1%.

Complicated, i.e. Progressive Massive Fibrosis (see Silicosis).

Complications (see Silicosis).

Cretinism (Congenital Hypothyroidism)

Appendicular Skeleton
1. Delayed appearance of ossification centres which may be (a) slightly granular, (b) finely stippled, (c) coarsely stippled or (d) fragmented. The femoral capital epiphyses may be divided into inner and outer halves.
2. Delayed epiphyseal closure.
3. Short long-bones with slender shafts, endosteal thickening and dense metaphyseal bands.
4. Coxa vara with shortened femoral neck and elevated greater trochanter.

Skull
1. Brachycephaly.
2. Multiple wormian bones.
3. Delayed development of vascular markings and diploic differentiation.
4. Delayed sutural closure.
5. Poorly developed sinuses and mastoids.

Axial Skeleton
1. Kyphosis at the thoracolumbar junction, usually associated with a hypoplastic or 'bullet-shaped' body of LV1 or LV2.

The bone changes may have completely regressed in adults.

Crohn's Disease

Colon and small bowel are affected equally. Gastric involvement is uncommon and is usually affected in continuity with disease in the duodenum. Oesophageal involvement is rare.

Small Bowel

1. Terminal ileum is the commonest site.
2. Asymmetrical involvement and skip lesions are characteristic. The disease predominates on the mesenteric border.
3. Apthoid ulcers — the earliest sign in the terminal ileum and colon.
4. Fissure ulcers — typically they are distributed in a longitudinal and transverse fashion. They may progress to abscess formation, sinuses and fistulae.
5. Blunting, thickening or distortion of the valvulae conniventes — the earliest sign in the small bowel proximal to the terminal ileum. Due to hyperplasia of lymphoid tissue producing an obstructive lymphoedema of the bowel wall.
6. 'Cobblestone' pattern — 2 possible causes
   (a) A combination of longitudinal and transverse fissure ulcers bounding intact mucosa. Or
   (b) The bulging of oedematous mucosal folds that are not closely attached to the underlying muscularis.
7. Separation of bowel loops — due to thickened bowel wall.
8. Strictures — which may be short or long, single or multiple. Significant clinical obstruction is less commonly observed.
9. Pseudosacculation.

Colon

1. Asymmetrical involvement and skip lesions. The rectum is involved in 30–50%.
2. Apthoid ulcers.
3. Deeper fissure ulcers which may produce a 'cobblestone' pattern.
4. Strictures.
5. Pseudosacculation.
6. Inflammatory pseudopolyps.
7. The ileocaecal valve may be thickened, narrowed and ulcerated.

Complications
1. Fistulae.
2. Perforation — which is usually localized and results in abscess formation.
3. Toxic megacolon.
4. Carcinoma
   (a) Colon — less common than in ulcerative colitis, but this may be because more patients with Crohn's disease undergo colectomy at an early stage.
   (b) Small bowel — 300× increased incidence.
5. Lymphoma.
6. Associated conditions
   (a) Erythema nodosum.
   (b) Arthritis
      (i) Spondyloarthritis mimicking ankylosing spondylitis. It follows a course independent of the bowel disease and precedes it in 25% of cases.
      (ii) Enteropathic synovitis, the activity of which parallels the bowel disease. The weight-bearing joints of the lower limbs, wrists and fingers are affected.
   (c) Cirrhosis.
   (d) Chronic active hepatitis.
   (e) Gallstones.
   (f) Oxalate urinary tract calculi.
   (g) Pericholangitis.
   (h) Cholangiocarcinoma.
   (i) Sclerosing cholangitis.

Cushing's Syndrome

Cushing's syndrome results from increased endogenous or exogenous cortisol.

Spontaneous Cushing's syndrome is rare and due to

Pituitary disease (Cushing's disease)	80%

  90% of these are due to adenoma and 20%
  have radiological evidence of an intrasellar
  tumour.

Adrenal disease — adenoma
　　　　　　 — carcinoma 　　　　　　　　　　 20%
Ectopic ACTH, e.g. from a carcinoma
　of the bronchus

Iatrogenic Cushing's syndrome is common and due to high doses of corticosteroids. The effects of excessive amounts of corticosteroids are:

1. Growth retardation in children.
2. Osteoporosis.
3. Pathological fractures which show excessive callus formation during healing; vertebral end-plate fractures, in particular, show prominent bone condensation.
4. Avascular necrosis of bone.
5. Increased incidence of infection — including osteomyelitis and septic arthritis (the knee is affected most frequently).
6. Hypertension.
7. Water retention resulting in oedema.

Cystic Fibrosis

An autosomal recessive condition in which the basic problem is one of excessively viscid mucus.

Cardiopulmonary
1. Bronchial wall thickening and mucus-filled bronchi.
2. Atelectasis — subsegmental, segmental or lobar (especially the right upper lobe).
3. Recurrent pneumonia.
4. Bronchiectasis.
5. Focal emphysema in generally overinflated lungs.
6. 'Honeycomb lung' (q.v.), ± pneumothorax (rare before puberty).
7. Low incidence of pleural effusion or empyema at all ages.
8. Cor pulmonale — more common in the older age group and often precedes death.

Gastrointestinal
1. Meconium ileus (10%), meconium peritonitis and meconium ileus equivalent (5–10%).
2. Thickened mucosal folds, nodular filling defects and small-bowel dilatation.

Liver
1. Hepatomegaly.
2. Portal hypertension.

Pancreas
1. Calcification (lithiasis).

Skeletal
1. Retarded maturation.
2. Clubbing and hypertrophic osteoarthropathy.

Sinuses
1. Chronic sinusitis — opaque maxillary antra in nearly all children over 2 years of age.
2. Nasal polyps (10–15%).
3. Mucocoele.

Down's Syndrome (Trisomy 21)

Craniofacial
1. Brachycephaly and microcephaly.
2. Hypoplasia of facial bones and sinuses.
3. Wide sutures and delayed closure. Multiple wormian bones.
4. Hypotelorism.
5. Underdeveloped teeth. No. 2| |2. Less caries than usual.

Axial Skeleton
1. Increased height and decreased AP diameter of lumbar vertebrae.
2. Atlantoaxial subluxation.
3. Incomplete fusion of vertebral arches of the lumbar spine.

Pelvis
1. Flared iliac wings with small acetabular angles resulting in an abnormal iliac index (iliac angle + acetabular angle).

Chest
1. Congenital heart disease (40%) — mainly endocardial cushion defects and aberrant right subclavian artery.
2. Eleven pairs of ribs.
3. Two ossification centres for the manubrium (90%).

Hands
1. Short tubular bones, clinodactyly (50%) and hypoplasia of the middle phalanx of the little finger (60%).

Gastrointestinal
1. Umbilical hernia.
2. Duodenal atresia or stenosis.
3. Tracheo-oesophageal fistula.
4. Anorectal anomalies.

Enchondroma

1. Age — 10–50 years.
2. Sites — hands and wrists predominate (50%). Any other bones formed in cartilage.
3. Appearances
   (a) Diaphyseal or diametaphyseal.
   (b) Well-defined lucency with a thin sclerotic rim.
   (c) Often expansile; cortex preserved.
   (d) Internal ground-glass appearance ± calcification.
   (e) Especially in long bones, may be multilocular.

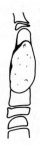

Syndromes
Ollier's disease — multiple enchondromata.
Maffucci's syndrome — enchondromata + haemangiomata.

Eosinophilic Granuloma

See 'Histiocytosis X'.

Ewing's Tumour

1. Age — 5–15 years
2. Sites — femur, pelvis and shoulder girdle.
3. Appearances
   (a) Diaphyseal or, less commonly, metaphyseal.
   (b) Ill-defined medullary destruction.
   (c) ± small areas of new bone formation.
   (d) Periosteal reaction — lamellated (onion skin), Codman's triangle or 'sunray' spiculation.
   (e) Soft-tissue extension.
   (f) Metastases to other bones and lungs.

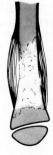

Extrinsic Allergic Alveolitis

An allergic reaction in the alveoli of sensitized individuals following repeated exposure to one of a number of specific antigens (see section 4.21).

Acute Exposure
1. Symptoms 4–8 hours after exposure (dyspnoea, dry cough, fever, malaise and myalgia).
2. The chest X-ray may be normal.
3. When radiological changes are present they usually parallel the severity of clinical symptoms. Changes consist of
   (a) Ground-glass, nodular or miliary shadows, 1–several mm in diameter, diffusely throughout both lungs but with some sparing of the apices and bases. Usually poorly defined.
   (b) Alveolar shadows, particularly in the lower zones, following heavy exposure to antigen.
   (c) Septal lines.
   (d) Hilar lymphadenopathy is rare but may be more frequent in mushroom-worker's lung.
4. Removal from antigen exposure results in resolution of the radiological changes over 1–several weeks.

Chronic Exposure
1. Persistent exposure to low doses of antigen.
2. The diffuse nodular pattern is replaced by the changes characteristic of diffuse interstitial fibrosis
   (a) Reticular pattern ⎫ but with
   (b) Loss of lung volume ⎬ marked upper-zone
   (c) 'Honeycomb' pattern ⎭ predominance.

Fibrous Dysplasia

Unknown pathogenesis. Medullary bone is replaced by fibrous tissue.

1. Diagnosis usually made between 3 and 15 years.
2. May be monostotic or polyostotic. In polyostotic cases the lesions tend to be unilateral; if bilateral then asymmetrical.
3. Most frequent sites are femur, pelvis, skull, mandible, ribs (most common cause of a focal expansile rib lesion) and humerus. Other bones are less frequently affected.
4. Radiological changes include
   (a) A cyst-like lesion in the diaphysis or metaphysis with endosteal scalloping ± bone expansion. No periosteal new bone. The epiphysis is only involved after fusion. Thick sclerotic border — 'rind' sign. Internally the lesion shows a ground-glass appearance ± irregular calcifications together with irregular sclerotic areas.
   (b) Bone deformity, e.g. shepherd's crook deformity of the proximal femur.
   (c) Growth disparity.
   (d) Accelerated bone maturation.
   (e) Skull shows mixed lucencies and sclerosis mainly on the convexity of the calvarium and the floor of the anterior fossa.
   (f) Leontiasis ossea is a sclerosing form affecting the face ± the skull base and producing leonine facies. In such cases extracranial lesions are rare. Involvement may be asymmetrical.
5. Associated endocrine abnormalities include
   (a) Sexual precocity (+ skin pigmentation) — in 30% of females with the polyostotic form. This constitutes the McCune–Albright syndrome.
   (b) Acromegaly, Cushing's syndrome, gynaecomastia and parathyroid hyperplasia (all rare).

Giant Cell Tumour

1. Age — 20–40 years (only 3% occur before epiphyseal closure).
2. Sites — long bones, distal femur especially; occasionally the sacrum or pelvis. Spine rarely.
3. Appearances
   (a) Epiphyseal and metaphyseal, i.e. subarticular.
   (b) A lucency with an ill-defined endosteal margin.
   (c) Eccentric expansion ± cortical destruction and soft-tissue extension.
   (d) Cortical ridges or internal septa produce a multilocular appearance.

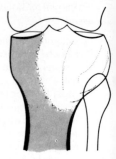

Gout

Caused by monosodium urate monohydrate or uric acid crystal deposition. Idiopathic (in the majority of patients) or associated with many other disorders, e.g. myeloproliferative diseases, drugs and chronic renal disease. Idiopathic gout may be divided into three stages

Asymptomatic Hyperuricaemia
1. No radiological signs but renal calculi or arthritis will develop in 20%.

Acute Gouty Arthritis
1. Mono- or oligoarticular; occasionally polyarticular.
2. Predilection for joints of the lower extremities, especially the 1st metatarsophalangeal joint (70%), intertarsal joints, ankles and knees. Other joints are affected in long-standing disease.
3. Soft-tissue swelling and joint effusion during the acute attack, with disappearance of the abnormalities as the attack subsides.

Chronic Tophaceous Gout

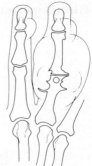

1. In 50% of patients with recurrent acute gout.
2. Eccentric, asymmetrical nodular deposits of calcium urate (tophi) in the synovium, subchondral bone, helix of the ear and in the soft tissues of the elbow, hand, foot, knee and forearm. Calcification of tophi is uncommon; ossification is rare.
3. Joint space is preserved until late in the disease.
4. Little or no osteoporosis until late, when there may be disuse osteoporosis.
5. Bony erosions are produced by tophaceous deposits and may be intra-articular, periarticular or well away from the joint. The latter two may be associated with an obvious soft-tissue mass. Erosions are round or oval, with the long axis in line with the bone. They may have a sclerotic margin. Some erosions have an overhanging lip of bone, which is strongly suggestive of the condition.
6. Severe erosive changes result in an arthritis mutilans.

Complications

1. Urolithiasis — in 10% of gout patients (higher in hot climates).
2. Renal disease
   (a) Acute urate nephropathy — precipitation of uric acid in the collecting ducts. Usually follows treatment with cytotoxic drugs.
   (b) Chronic urate nephropathy — rare.

Haemangioma

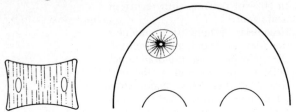

1. Age — 10–50 years
2. Sites — vertebra (dorsal lumbar) or skull vault.
3. Appearances
   (a) Vertebra — coarse vertical striations, usually affecting only the body but the appendages are, uncommonly, also involved.
   (b) Skull — radial spiculation ('sunburst') within a well-defined vault lucency. 'Hair-on-end' appearance in tangential views.

Haemochromatosis

A genetically determined primary abnormality of iron metabolism. Also occurs secondary to alcoholic cirrhosis or multiple blood transfusions, e.g. in thalassaemia or chronic excessive oral iron ingestion.

Clinically — cirrhosis, skin pigmentation, diabetes (bronze diabetics), arthropathy and, later, ascites and cardiac failure.

Bones and Joints

1. Osteoporosis.
2. Chondrocalcinosis — due to calcium pyrophosphate dihydrate deposition (q.v.).
3. Arthropathy — resembles the arthropathy of calcium pyrophosphate deposition disease (q.v.), but shows a predilection for the metacarpophalangeal joints (especially the 2nd and 3rd), the midcarpal joints and the carpometacarpal joints. It also exhibits distinctive beak-like osteophytes and is less rapidly progressive.

Liver and Spleen

1. Mottled increased density of liver and spleen due to the deposition of iron.

Haemophilia

Classical (Factor VIII deficiency) or Christmas disease (Factor IX deficiency). Both are X-linked recessive traits, i.e. manifest in males and carried by females.

Joints
1. Knee, elbow, ankle, hip and shoulder are most frequently affected.
2. Soft-tissue swelling due to haemarthrosis which may appear to be unusually dense owing to the presence of haemosiderin in the chronically thickened synovium.
3. Periarticular osteoporosis.
4. Erosion of articular surfaces, with subchondral cysts.
5. Preservation of joint space until late.
6. Accelerated maturation and growth of epiphyses resulting in disparity of size between epiphysis and diaphysis.
7. Contractures.

Bones
1. Osteonecrosis — especially in the femoral head and talus.
2. Haemophilic pseudotumour — in the ilium, femur and tibia most frequently
   (a) Intraosseous — a well-defined medullary lucency with a sclerotic margin. It may breach the cortex. ± periosteal reaction and soft-tissue component.
   (b) Subperiosteal — periosteal reaction with pressure resorption of the cortex and a soft-tissue mass.
3. Fractures — secondary to osteoporosis.

Soft Tissues
1. Pseudotumour — slow growing.
2. Ectopic ossification.

Further Reading
Stoker D.J. & Murray R.O. (1974) Skeletal changes in haemophilia and other bleeding disorders. *Semin. Roentgenol.*, 9: 185–93.

Histiocytosis X

A disease characterized by intense proliferation of reticulo-histiocytic elements. Younger patients have more disseminated disease. There are three clinical subgroups.

Eosinophilic Granuloma
1. Accounts for 50% of histiocytosis.
2. Commonest in 4–7 year olds, who present with bone pain, local swelling and irritability.
3. 50–75% have solitary lesions. When multiple, usually only two or three. Long bones, pelvis, skull and flat bones are the most common sites involved.
4. Radiological changes in the skeleton include
   (a) Well-defined lucency in the medulla ± thin sclerotic rim. ± endosteal scalloping. True expansion is uncommon except in ribs and vertebral bodies. ± overlying periosteal reaction.
   (b) Multilocular lucency, without expansion, in the pelvis.
   (c) Punched-out lucencies in the skull vault with little or no surrounding sclerosis. May coalesce to give a 'geographical skull'.
   (d) Destructive lesions in the skull base, mastoids, sella or mandible ('floating teeth').
   (e) Vertebra plana, with intact intervertebral discs.
5. Lung involvement in < 10% and associated with a worse prognosis.
   (a) Hilar lymphadenopathy.
   (b) Miliary shadowing.
   (c) 'Honeycomb lung'.

Hand–Schüller–Christian Disease
1. Commonest in 1–3 year olds.
2. Osseous lesions together with mild to moderate visceral involvement which includes lymphadenopathy, hepato-splenomegaly, skin lesions, diabetes insipidus, exophthalmos and pulmonary disease.
3. Bone lesions are similar to eosinophilic granuloma, but more numerous and widely distributed.

Letterer–Siwe Disease
1. Major visceral involvement with less prominent bone involvement during the first year of life.
2. Bone lesions are poorly defined.

Homocystinuria

An autosomal recessive inborn error of metabolism. A lack of cystathionine synthetase results in the accumulation of homocystine and methionine, with a deficiency of cystathionine and cystine.

1. Mental defect (60%).
2. Tall stature, slim build and arachnodactyly, with a morphological resemblance to Marfan's syndrome.
3. Pectus excavatum or carinatum, kyphoscoliosis, genu valgum and pes cavus.
4. Osteoporosis.
5. Medial degeneration of the aorta and elastic arteries.
6. Arterial and venous thromboses.
7. Lens subluxation — usually downward.

Hurler's Syndrome

A mucopolysaccharidosis transmitted as an autosomal recessive trait. Clinical features become evident at the end of the first year — dwarfism, mental retardation, coarse facial features, corneal opacification, deformed teeth and hepatosplenomegaly. Respiratory infections and cardiac failure usually lead to death in the first decade.

Craniofacial
1. Scaphocephalic macrocephaly.
2. ± hydrocephalus.
3. J-shaped sella (prominent sulcus chiasmatus).

Axial Skeleton
1. Oval vertebral bodies with an antero-inferior beak.
2. Kyphosis and a thoracolumbar gibbus.
3. Posterior scalloping with widened interpedicular distance.
4. Short neck.

Appendicular Skeleton
1. Thickened diaphyses.
2. Angulated, oblique growth plates, e.g. those of the distal radius and ulna are angled toward each other.
3. Coxa valga (common). Genu valgum (always).
4. Trident hands with a coarse trabecular pattern. Proximal tapering of metacarpals.

Cardiovascular System
1. Cardiac failure due to intimal thickening of coronary arteries or valves.

N.B. Hunter's syndrome is very similar clinically and radiologically, but the differences are:
(a) X-linked recessive transmission (i.e. no affected females).
(b) Later onset (2–6 yrs) and slower progression (death in the 2nd or 3rd decade).
(c) No corneal clouding.

Hyperparathyroidism, Primary

Causes
1. Adenoma of one gland (90%). (2% of adenomas are multiple.)
2. Hyperplasia of all four glands (5%). (More likely if there is a family history.)
3. Carcinoma of one gland.
4. Ectopic parathormone — e.g. from a carcinoma of the bronchus.
5. Multiple endocrine adenopathy syndrome (type 1) — hyperplasia or adenoma associated with pituitary adenoma and pancreatic tumour.

Bones
1. Osteopenia — uncommon. When advanced there is loss of the fine trabeculae and sometimes a ground-glass appearance.
2. Subperiosteal bone resorption — particularly affecting the radial side of the middle phalanx of the middle finger, medial proximal tibia, lateral and occasionally medial end of clavicle, symphysis pubis, ischial tuberosity, medial femoral neck, dorsum sellae, superior surface of ribs and proximal humerus. Severe disease produces terminal phalangeal resorption and, in children, the 'rotting fence-post' appearance of the proximal femur.
3. Diffuse cortical change — cortical tunnelling eventually leading to a 'basketwork' appearance. 'Pepper-pot skull'.
4. Brown tumours — the solitary sign in 3% of cases. Most frequent in the mandible, ribs, pelvis and femora.
5. Bone softening — basilar invagination, wedged or codfish vertebrae, kyphoscoliosis, triradiate pelvis. Pathological fractures.

Soft Tissues
1. Calcification in soft tissues, pancreas, lung and arteries.

Joints
1. Marginal erosions — predominantly the distal interphalangeal joints, the ulnar side of the base of the little-finger metacarpal and the hamate. No joint-space narrowing.
2. Weakened subarticular bone, leading to collapse.
3. Chondrocalcinosis (calcium pyrophosphate dihydrate deposition disease) and true gout.
4. Periarticular calcification, including capsular and tendon calcification.

Kidney
1. Nephrocalcinosis.
2. Calculi (in 50%).

Hypercalcaemia
1. Asymptomatic (in 15%) or overt (in 8%).

Gastrointestinal Tract
1. Peptic ulcer.
2. Pancreatitis.

Hypoparathyroidism

1. Short stature, dry skin, alopecia, tetany ± mental retardation.
2. Skeletal changes affecting the entire skeleton.
3. Minimal, generalized increased density of the skeleton, but especially affecting the metaphyses.
4. Calcification of paraspinal ligaments (secondary to elevation of plasma phosphate, which combines with calcium, resulting in heterotopic calcium phosphate deposits).
5. Basal ganglia calcification — uncommon.

Hypophosphatasia

Autosomal recessive. Deficiency of serum and tissue alkaline phosphatase, with excessive urinary excretion of phosphoethanolamine. 50% die in early infancy.

Neonatal Form
1. Most severely affected. Stillborn or die within 6 months.
2. Clinically — hypotonia, irritability, vomiting respiratory insufficiency, failure to thrive, convulsions and small stature with bowed legs.
3. Radiologically
   (a) Profoundly deficient mineralization with increased liability to fractures.
   (b) Irregular lack of metaphyseal mineralization affecting especially the wrists, knees and costochondral junctions.

Infantile Form
1. Initially asymptomatic, but between 2 weeks and 6 months shows the same symptoms as the neonatal form. Most survive.
2. Radiologically
   (a) Cupped and frayed metaphyses with widened growth-plates.
   (b) Demineralized epiphyses.
   (c) Defective mineralization of skull, including sutures which appear widened.
   (d) Premature sutural fusion → craniostenosis with brachycephaly.

Childhood Form
1. Presents 6 months – 2 years with bowed legs, genu valgum, delayed walking, bone pain, dental caries and premature loss of teeth.
2. Radiologically
   (a) Mild rickets.
   (b) No craniostenosis.

Adult Form
1. Osteomalácia — both clinically and radiologically.

Hypothyroidism

See 'Cretinism'.

Juvenile Chronic Arthritis

Three main clinical subgroups account for 70% of cases

Systemic Onset
1. Most common at 1–5 years. M = F.
2. Severe extra-articular clinical manifestations include pyrexia, rash, lymphadenopathy and hepatosplenomegaly.
3. Joint involvement is late, but eventually a polyarthritis affects especially the knees, wrists, carpi, ankles and tarsi.

Polyarticular Onset
1. Onset at any age. More common in females.
2. Arthritis predominates with a similar distribution to the systemic onset, but also including the small joints of the fingers and toes. The cervical spine is involved frequently and early.
3. Prolonged disease leads to growth retardation and abnormal epiphyseal development.

Pauciarticular or Monoarticular Onset (most common presentation)
1. Most commonly presents at 1–5 years.
2. Four or less joints involved at the onset — knees, ankles and hips most commonly.
3. ± iridocyclitis.

Less Common Chronic Arthritides in Children
1. Seropositive juvenile onset rheumatoid arthritis — closely resembles the adult disease. Most common over 10 years of age and more common in girls.
2. Juvenile ankylosing spondylitis.
3. Juvenile psoriatic arthritis.
4. Enteropathic arthritis.

Radiological Changes

1. Periarticular soft-tissue swelling.
2. Osteopenia — juxta-articular, diffuse or band-like in the metaphyses; the latter particularly in the distal femur, proximal tibia, distal radius and distal tibia.
3. Accelerated bone growth with large epiphyses and early fusion of growth-plates.
4. Over- or undergrowth of diaphyses.
5. Periostitis — common. Mainly periarticular in the phalanges, metacarpals and metatarsals, but when diaphyseal will eventually result in enlarged rectangular tubular bones.
6. Erosions and joint-space narrowing are late manifestations.
7. Epiphyseal compression fractures.
8. Subluxation and dislocation — most commonly in the hip leading to protrusio acetabuli. Atlanto-axial subluxation is most frequent in seropositive juvenile onset rheumatoid arthritis.
9. Bony ankylosis — especially in the carpus and tarsus.

Lymphoma

Intrathoracic Lymphadenopathy

1. 66% of patients with Hodgkin's disease have intrathoracic disease and 99% of these have intrathoracic lymphadeno-pathy.
2. 40% of patients with non-Hodgkin's lymphoma have intrathoracic disease and 90% of these have intrathoracic lymphadenopathy.
3. Nodes involved are (in order of frequency) anterior mediastinal, paratracheal, tracheobronchial, bronchopul-monary and subcarinal. Involvement tends to be bilateral and asymmetrical, although unilateral disease is not uncommon.
4. Nodes show a rapid response to radiotherapy and 'eggshell' calcification of lymphnodes may be observed following radiotherapy.

Pulmonary Disease

1. More common in Hodgkin's disease than non-Hodgkin's lymphoma.
2. Very unusual without lymphadenopathy, but may be the first evidence of recurrence after radiotherapy.
3. Most frequently one or more large opacities with an irregular outline. ± air bronchogram.
4. Collapse due to endobronchial lymphoma or, less fre-quently, extrinsic compression. (Collapse is less common than in bronchial carcinoma.)
5. Lymphatic obstruction → oedema or lymphangitis carci-nomatosa.
6. Miliary or larger opacities widely disseminated through-out the lungs.
7. Cavitation — eccentrically within a mass and with a thick wall. (More common than in bronchial carcinoma.)
8. Calcification following radiotherapy.
9. Soft-tissue mass adjacent to a rib deposit.
10. Pleural and pericardial effusions.

Gastrointestinal Tract

Involvement may be the primary presentation (5% of all lymphomas) or be a part of generalized disease (50% at autopsy). In descending order of frequency, the stomach, small intestine, rectum and colon may be involved.

Stomach

1. Primary lymphoma accounts for 2.5% of all gastric neoplasms and 2.5% of lymphomas present with a stomach lesion. Non-Hodgkin's lymphoma accounts for 80%.
2. The radiological manifestations comprise
   (a) Diffuse mucosal thickening and irregularity ± decreased distensibility and peristaltic activity. ± multiple ulcers.
   (b) Smooth nodular mass ± central ulceration. Surrounding mucosa may be normal or show thickened folds.
   (c) Single or multiple ulcers with irregular margins.
   (d) Thickening of the wall with narrowing of the lumen. If the distal stomach is involved there may be extension into the duodenum.
   (e) Duodenal ulcer associated with a gastric mass.

Small Intestine

1. Usually secondary to contiguous spread from mesenteric lymph nodes. Primary disease only in non-Hodgkin's lymphoma.
2. Usually more than one of the following signs is evident
   (a) Irregular mucosal infiltration → thick folds ± nodularity.
   (b) Irregular polypoid mass ± barium tracts within it or central ulceration.
   (c) Annular constriction — usually a long segment.
   (d) Aneurysmal dilatation, with no internal mucosal pattern.
   (e) Polyps — multiple and small or solitary and large. The latter may induce an intussusception.
   (f) Multiple ulcers.
   (g) Non-specific malabsorption pattern.
   (h) Fistula.
   (i) Perforation.

Colon and Rectum
1. Rarely involved. Caecum and rectum more frequently involved than the rest of the colon.
2. Radiologically the disease may show
   (a) Polypoidal mass — which may induce an intussusception.
   (b) Diffuse infiltration of the wall.
   (c) Constricting annular lesion.

Retroperitoneal Lymphadenopathy
1. The typical lymphographic appearances are
   (a) Enlarged nodes.
   (b) Foamy or 'ghost-like' internal architectural pattern.
   (c) Discrete filling defects.
   (d) Non-filling of lymph nodes.

Skeleton
1. Radiological involvement in 10–20% of patients with Hodgkin's disease (50% at autopsy).
2. Involvement arises either from direct spread from contiguous lymph nodes or infiltration of bone marrow (spine, pelvis, major long bones, thoracic cage and skull are sites of predilection).
3. Patterns of bone involvement are
   (a) Predominantly osteolytic.
   (b) Mixed lytic and sclerotic.
   (c) Predominantly sclerotic — de novo or following radiotherapy to a lytic lesion.
   (d) 'Moth-eaten' — characteristic of round cell malignancies.
4. In addition the spine may show
   (a) Anterior erosion of a vertebral body due to involvement of an adjacent paravertebral lymph node.
   (b) Solitary dense vertebral body (ivory vertebra).
5. Hypertrophic osteoarthropathy.

Central Nervous System
1. Primary lymphoma of brain (microgliomatosis) accounts for 1% of brain tumours.
2. The cerebrum, brainstem and cerebellum are affected (in order of frequency).
3. Two patterns may be recognized at CT
   (a) Large round or oval space-occupying lesion showing increased attenuation and surrounding oedema. Marked homogeneous enhancement (although avascular at angiography). Multifocal in 50%.
   (b) Cuff of tissue around the lateral ventricles with marked enhancement.

Further Reading

Craig O. & Gregson R. (1981). Primary lymphoma of the gastrointestinal tract. *Clin. Radiol.*, 32: 63–71.
Felson B. (ed.) (1980) The lymphomas and leukaemias. Part 1. *Semin. Roentgenol.*, 15(3).
Felson B. (ed.) (1980) The lymphomas and leukaemias. Part 2. *Semin. Roentgenol.*, 15(4).
Privett J.T.J., Rhys Davies E. & Roylance J. (1977). The radiological features of gastric lymphoma. *Clin. Radiol.*, 28: 457–63.
Strickland B. (1967). Intrathoracic Hodgkin's disease. Part II. Peripheral manifestations of Hodgkin's disease in the chest. *Br. J. Radiol.*, 40: 930–8.
Thomson J.C.G. & Brownell B. (1981) Computed tomographic appearances in microgliomatosis. *Clin. Radiol.*, 32: 367–74.

Marfan's Syndrome

A connective tissue disorder transmitted as an autosomal dominant trait, but with extremely variable expression.

1. Tall stature, long slim limbs and arachnodactyly.
2. Joint laxity.
3. Scoliosis (60%) and kyphosis.
4. Pectus excavatum or carinatum.
5. Narrow facies with a narrow, high arched palate.
6. Lens subluxation — usually upwards.
7. Ascending aortic dilatation ± dissection. Less commonly aneurysms of the descending thoracic or abdominal aorta or pulmonary artery.

Morquio's Syndrome

A mucopolysaccharidosis transmitted as an autosomal recessive trait. Clinical presentation during the second year, with decreased growth, progressive skeletal deformity, corneal opacities, lymphadenopathy, cardiac lesions and deafness.

Axial Skeleton
1. Universal vertebra plana. Wide discs.
2. Hypoplastic dens.
3. Hypoplastic dorsolumbar vertebra which may be displaced posteriorly.
4. Central anterior vertebral body beaks.
5. Short neck.
6. Dorsal scoliosis and dorsolumbar kyphosis.

Appendicular Skeleton
1. Defective irregular ossification of the femoral capital epiphyses leading to flattening.
2. Genu valgum.
3. Short, wide tubular bones with irregular metaphyses. Proximal tapering of the metacarpals.
4. Irregular carpal and tarsal bones.

Cardiovascular System
1. Late onset aortic regurgitation.

Multiple Myeloma/Plasmacytoma

Plasma cell neoplasms of bone are solitary (plasmacytoma; 3% of all plasma cell tumours) or multiple (multiple myeloma; 94% of all plasma cell tumours). 3% of all plasma cell tumours are solely extraskeletal.

Plasmacytoma
1. A well-defined, grossly expansile bone lesion arising, most commonly, in the spine, pelvis or ribs.
2. It may also exhibit soft-tissue extension, internal septa or pathological fracture.

Multiple Myeloma
Radiological manifestations are skeletal and extraskeletal.

SKELETAL
1. 80–90% have an abnormal skeleton at the time of diagnosis.
2. The skeleton may
   (a) be normal — uncommon;
   (b) show generalized osteopenia only — rare;
   (c) show osteopenia with discrete lucencies
      (i) The lucencies are usually
         — widely disseminated at the time of diagnosis (spine, pelvis, skull, ribs and shafts of long bones);
         — uniform in size (c.f. metastases, which are usually of varying size);
         — well-defined, with a narrow zone of transition.
      (ii) Vertebral body collapse, occasionally with disc destruction. ± paravertebral shadow. Involvement of pedicles is late.
      (iii) Rib lesions tend to be expansile and associated with extrapleural soft-tissue masses.
      (iv) Pathological fractures occur and healing is accompanied by much callus.
   (d) show a permeating, mottled pattern of bone destruction similar to other round cell malignancies, e.g. Ewing's sarcoma, anaplastic metastatic carcinoma, leukaemia and reticulum cell sarcoma.
   (e) show multiple sclerotic lesions which mimic osteoblastic metastases (2%).

EXTRASKELETAL
1. Hypercalcaemia (30%).
2. Soft-tissue tumours in sinuses, the submucosa of the pharynx and trachea, cervical lymph nodes, skin and gastrointestinal tract.
3. Hepatosplenomegaly.

Further Reading

Meszaros W.T. (1974) The many facets of multiple myeloma. *Semin. Roentgenol.*, 9: 219–28.

Neurofibromatosis

Autosomal dominant but 50% are spontaneous mutations.

Skull and Brain
1. Hemihypertrophy or hemiatrophy of the cranium. Macro-cranium.
2. Dysplastic sphenoid — absent greater wing ± lesser wing (empty orbit), absent posterolateral wall of the orbit. May produce proptosis.
3. Lytic defects in the calvarium, especially in or near the lambdoid suture.
4. Optic nerve gliomas (common). Optic nerve sheath meningiomas (rare).
5. Neuromas, especially acoustic neuromas. If bilateral they are virtually pathognomonic of the condition.
6. Meningiomas.
7. Heavy calcification of the choroid plexuses is rare but classical.

Thorax
1. Rib notching, 'twisted ribbon' ribs and splaying of ribs.
2. Interstitial pulmonary fibrosis progressing to a 'honey-comb lung'.

Axial Skeleton
1. Sharp angular kyphoscoliosis (in 10%) with dysplastic vertebral bodies.
2. Posterior scalloping due to dural ectasia.
3. Enlarged intervertebral foramina and eccentric unilateral scalloping due to localized neurofibromas.

Appendicular Skeleton
1. Overgrowth or, less commonly, undergrowth of long bones.
2. Overtubulation or undertubulation (due to cortical thickening).
3. Anterior and lateral bowing of the tibia is common and is usually evident in the first year. It frequently progresses to —
4. Pseudarthrosis.
5. Intraosseous neurofibromas present as subperiosteal or cortical lucencies with a smooth expanded outer margin.
6. Cortical pressure resorption from an adjacent soft-tissue neurofibroma.
7. Cortical defects may also be due to dysplastic periosteum.

Other
1. Soft-tissue tumours.
2. Renal artery stenosis or aneurysm.
3. Phaeochromocytoma (in 1%).

Further Reading
Klatte E.C., Franken E.A. & Smith J.A. (1976). The radiographic spectrum in neurofibromatosis. *Semin. Roentgenol.*, 11: 17–33.

Neuropathic Arthropathy

Disease	Sites of involvement
Diabetes mellitus	Metatarsophalangeal, tarsometatarsal and intertarsal joints
Steroid treatment	Hip and knee
Syringomyelia	Shoulder, elbow, wrist and cervical spine
Tabes dorsalis	Knee, hip, ankle and lumbar spine
Congenital insensitivity to pain	Ankle and intertarsal joints
Myelomeningocoele	Ankle and intertarsal joints
Leprosy	Hands (interphalangeal), feet (metatarsophalangeal) and lower limbs
Chronic alcoholism	Metatarsophalangeal and interphalangeal joints

Radiological changes include
1. Variable progression, but often rapid. In the early stages can resemble osteoarthritis.
2. Joint effusion.
3. Osteochondral fractures and fragmentation of articular surfaces.
4. Intra-articular bony debris.
5. Excessive callus formation.
6. Subluxations and dislocations.
7. Bone density is normal but in diabetes and syringomyelia superadded infection is not uncommon, resulting in juxta-articular osteoporosis.
8. Bone resorption can produce a 'cup and pencil' appearance.

Non-accidental Injury (Battered-Child Syndrome)

Skeletal
1. Fractures in over 50% of cases. 25% of these have multiple fractures, characteristically at different stages of healing.
2. Commonest sites are (in order of frequency) ribs, humerus, femur, tibia and skull.
3. Shaft fractures are twice as common as metaphyseal fractures, although the latter are characteristic.
4. Metaphyseal fractures result from avulsion of fragments of the metaphysis, by the pull of strongly anchored periosteum. Small segments or complete rims of bone (bucket handle fractures) can be avulsed.
5. Skull fractures in 20%.
6. Subperiosteal bleeding leads to periosteal reaction and will eventually ossify. If there is repeated trauma or inadequate immobilization the periosteal reaction can be massive.

Extraskeletal
1. Intracranial haemorrhage — subdural, extradural or intracerebral.
2. Cerebral oedema.
3. Haematoma and laceration of any intra-abdominal viscus.
4. Pulmonary contusion.

Further Reading
Cameron J.M. & Rae L.J. (1975) *Atlas of the Battered Child Syndrome*. Edinburgh: Churchill Livingstone.

Non-ossifying Fibroma (Fibrous Cortical Defect)

1. Age — 10–20 years.
2. Sites — femur and tibia.
3. Appearances
   (a) Diametaphyseal, becoming diaphysael as the bone grows.
   (b) Well-defined lucency with a sclerotic margin.
   (c) Eccentric ± slight expansion; in thin bones, e.g. fibula, it occupies the entire width of the bone.

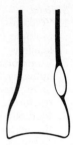

Ochronosis

See 'Alkaptonuria'.

Osteoblastoma

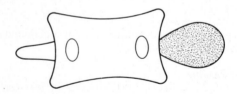

1. Age — 10–20 years.
2. Sites — vertebra (neural arch predominantly) and, less commonly, in the long bones.
3. Appearances
   (a) Well-defined lucency with a sclerotic rim.
   (b) May be expansile, but the cortex is preserved.
   (c) ± internal calcification.
   (d) May be purely sclerotic in the spine.
   (e) In long bones it is metaphyseal or diaphyseal.

Osteochondroma (Exostosis)

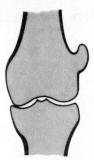

1. Age — 10–20 years.
2. Sites — distal femur, proximal tibia, proximal humerus, pelvis and scapula. When there are multiple osteochondromata the condition is termed diaphyseal aclasis.
3. Appearances
   (a) Metaphyseal.
   (b) Well-defined eccentric protrusion with the parent cortex and trabeculae continuous with that of the tumour.
   (c) Tumour is usually directed away from the end of the bone and migrates away from the end as growth proceeds.
   (d) The cartilage cap is not visible in childhood, but becomes calcified in the adult.
   (e) If large → failure of correct modelling.
   (f) Rapid growth of a stable lesion suggests transformation to a chondrosarcoma (less than 1% of cases).

Osteogenesis Imperfecta

A generalized mesenchymal disorder. Autosomal dominant.

1. Three clinical types.
   (a) Infantile — if severe, the child is stillborn.
   (b) Intermediate — appearing shortly after the child begins to walk.
   (c) Tarda — diagnosed in adulthood and relatively uncommon.
2. Blue sclerae; deafness due to otosclerosis.
3. Generalized osteoporosis with cortical thinning.
4. Multiple fractures which heal with exuberant callus. Compression fractures of vertebral bodies.
5. Bone softening — bowed long bones, acetabular protrusion with infolding of the lateral walls of the pelvis, codfish vertebrae and basilar impression.
6. Wormian bones.

Osteogenic Sarcoma

1. Age — 10–25 years with a second peak in the 7th decade (flat bones).
2. Sites — distal femur, proximal tibia, proximal humerus and pelvis.
3. Predisposing factors — Paget's disease, irradiation, osteochondroma, ? fibrous dysplasia and ?? osteogenesis imperfecta.
4. Appearances
   (a) Metaphyseal.
   (b) May be predominantly lytic, sclerotic or mixed.
   (c) Wide zone of transition with normal bone.
   (d) Cortical destruction with soft-tissue extension.
   (e) ± Internal calcification of bone.
   (f) Periosteal reaction — 'sunray' spiculation, lamellated and/or Codman's triangle.

Osteoid Osteoma

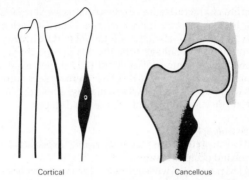

Cortical   Cancellous

1. Age — 10–30 years.
2. Sites — most commonly femur and tibia.
3. Appearances

   Cortical
   (a) Central lucent nidus (less than 1 cm) ± dense calcified centre.
   (b) Dense surrounding bone.
   (c) Eccentric bone expansion ± periosteal reaction.

   Cancellous
   (a) Usually femoral neck.
   (b) Lucent lesion with bone sclerosis a distance away. The head and neck may be osteoporotic.

Osteomalacia

Increased uncalcified osteoid in the mature skeleton.

1. Decreased bone density.
2. Looser's zones — bilaterally symmetrical transverse lucent bands of uncalcified osteoid which, later in the disease, have sclerotic margins. Common sites are the scapulae, femoral necks and shafts, pubic rami and ribs.
3. Coarsening of the trabecular pattern with ill-defined trabeculae.
4. Bone softening — protrusio acetabulae, bowing of long bones, biconcave vertebral bodies and basilar invagination.

Paget's Disease

A condition characterized by excessive abnormal remodelling of bone. Increasing prevalence with age — rare in patients less than 40 years old, 3% of the population in middle age and 10% of the population in old age. The disease predominates in the axial skeleton — spine (75%), skull (65%), pelvis (40%) — and proximal femur (75%). (The percentages represent patients with Paget's disease in whom these sites are affected.) Monostotic disease does occur. There are 3 stages

Active (Osteolytic)
1. Skull — osteoporosis circumscripta, especially in the frontal and occipital bones.
2. Long bones — a well-defined, advancing radiolucency with a V-shaped margin which begins subarticularly.

Osteolytic and Osteosclerotic
1. Skull — osteoporosis circumscripta with focal areas of bone sclerosis.
2. Pelvis — mixed osteolytic and osteosclerotic areas.
3. Long bones — epiphyseal and metaphyseal sclerosis with diaphyseal lucency.

Inactive (Osteosclerotic)
1. Skull — thickened vault. 'Cotton wool' areas of sclerotic bone. The facial bones are not commonly affected (c.f. fibrous dysplasia).
2. Spine — especially the lumbar spine. Enlargement of vertebrae and coarsened trabeculae. Cortical thickening produces the 'picture frame' vertebral body. Ivory vertebra.
3. Pelvis — widening and coarsened trabeculation of the pelvic ring, with splitting of the iliopectineal line may progress to widespread changes in the pelvis which are commonly asymmetrical.
4. Long bones — sclerosis due to coarsened, thickened trabeculae. Cortical thickening with encroachment on the medullary canal. The epiphyseal region is nearly always involved.

Complications
1. Bone softening — bowed bones, basilar invagination and protrusio acetabuli.
2. Fractures — transverse with a predilection for the convex aspect of the bone and which usually only partially traverse the bone.
3. Sarcomatous change — in 1% of patients (5–10% if there is widespread involvement). Femur, pelvis and humerus most commonly affected. Osteogenic sarcoma (50%), fibrosarcoma (25%) and chondrosarcoma (10%) are the most common histological diagnoses. They are predominantly lytic.
4. Degenerative joint disease — most frequent in the hip and knee.
5. Neurological complications — nerve entrapment and spinal-cord compression.
6. High output cardiac failure.
7. Extramedullary haemopoiesis.
8. Osteomyelitis.

Plasmacytoma

See 'Multiple myeloma/plasmacytoma'.

Polycystic Disease, Infantile

Autosomal recessive trait. Polycystic kidneys, with periportal hepatic fibrosis and bile duct obstruction.

Polycystic Disease of the Newborn
1. Presents in the first few days with renal failure and/or respiratory distress because of elevated diaphragms. Majority die in a few days.
2. Bilateral large smooth kidneys with dense striated nephrograms (because of dilated tubules).
3. Calyces are not usually demonstrated but are normal.

Polycystic Disease of Childhood
1. Presents at 3–5 years.
2. Renal cysts are less prominent and hepatic fibrosis is greater. Presentation is, therefore, with portal hyptertension.
3. Kidneys may be similar to the newborn type (although not so massive) or to the adult type. Multiple hepatic cysts.

Polycystic Disease, Adult

Autosomal dominant trait. Presents in 3rd–4th decade and terminal renal failure occurs within 10 years.

Kidneys

1. Bilateral, but asymmetrical, enlarged lobulated kidneys. Unilateral in 8%.
2. Miltiple smooth defects in the nephrogram with elongation and deformity of calyces giving a 'spider leg' appearance. Cysts may produce filling defects in the renai pelvis. ± calcification in cyst walls.
3. Increased incidence of renal cell carcinoma (may be bilateral).

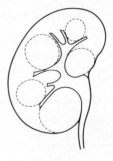

Other Organs

1. Cystic changes in the liver (in 30%) and, less commonly, in the pancreas and spleen.
2. Displacement of bowel.
3. Intracranial aneurysms in 10%.

Pseudohypoparathyroidism

End organ unresponsiveness to parathormone. X-linked dominant transmission.

1. Short stature, round face, thickset features, mental retardation and hypocalcaemia.
2. Short 4th and 5th metacarpals and metatarsals.
3. Basal ganglia calcification (50%).
4. Soft-tissue calcification.

Pseudopseudohypoparathyroidism

Similar clinical and radiological features to pseudohypoparathyroidism but with a normal plasma calcium.

Psoriatic Arthropathy

Occurs in 5% of psoriatics and may antedate the skin changes. There are five clinical and radiological types.

1. Polyarthritis with predominant involvement of the distal interphalangeal joints.
2. Seronegative polyarthritis simulating rheumatoid arthritis.
3. Monoarthritis or asymmetrical oligoarthritis.
4. Spondyloarthritis which can mimic ankylosing spondylitis.
5. Arthritis mutilans (commonly associated with severe skin changes).

The radiological changes comprise

1. Involvement of synovial and cartilaginous joints and entheses.
2. Joints most frequently affected are the interphalangeal joints of the hands and feet, the metacarpophalangeal and metatarsophalangeal joints, the sacro-iliac joints and those in the spine. The large joints are relatively spared. Involvement is asymmetrical.
3. Preserved bone density.
4. Soft-tissue swelling — periarticular or fusiform of a digit.
5. The joint space is narrowed in the large joints and widened in the small joints because of severe destruction of subchondral bone.
6. Erosions which are initially periarticular and progress to involve the entire articular surface. 'Cup and pencil' deformity. Severe destructive changes result in an arthritis mutilans. Erosions also occur at entheses.
7. Bony proliferation (a) adjacent to the erosions and (b) at tendon and ligament insertions.
8. Periosteal new bone — particularly in the hands and feet.
9. Ankylosis — especially at the interphalangeal joints of the hands and feet.
10. Distal phalangeal tuft resorption — almost always with severe nail changes.
11. Sacro-iliitis and spondylitis with paravertebral ossification.

Pulmonary Embolic Disease

Clinical conditions which predispose to venous thromboembolism are

1. Surgical procedures, especially major abdominal and gynaecological surgery and hip operations.
2. Trauma.
3. Prolonged bed-rest.
4. Neoplastic disease.
5. Pregnancy and the puerperium.
6. Oestrogens.

Pulmonary embolism is massive if more than 50% of the major pulmonary arteries are involved and minor if less than 50% are involved. Duration of embolism in the pulmonary arteries may be acute (< 48 hours), subacute (several days or weeks) or chronic (months or years).

Acute or Subacute Massive Embolism
1. The chest X-ray is most commonly normal.
2. Asymmetrical oligaemia — often best diagnosed by comparison with a previous chest X-ray. The main pulmonary artery may be enlarged.

Acute Minor
1. Although segmental oligaemia ± dilatation of the segmental artery proximal to the obstruction may be observed, this is uncommon and the chest X-ray is often normal.
2. Pulmonary infarction follows in about 33%. The signs are non-specific but include
   (a) Subpleural consolidation — segmental or subsegmental. Single or multiple.
   (b) Segmental collapse and later linear (plate) atelectasis.
   (c) Pleural reaction with a small effusion.
   (d) Elevation of the hemidiaphragm on the affected side.
   (e) Cavitation of the infarct.

3. Infarction is more common on the right side and in the lower zones.

N.B. The ventilation–perfusion radionuclide lung-scan is an extremely useful investigation for the diagnosis of pulmonary embolism, especially as the chest X-ray is so commonly normal. The characteristic abnormality is a segmental perfusion defect at the periphery of the lung with no corresponding ventilation defect, i.e. a mismatched defect. This is pathognomonic of pulmonary embolism. When the chest X-ray shows collapse or infarction the lung scan shows a corresponding ventilation and perfusion defect, i.e. a matched defect. This is a non-specific finding seen with any pulmonary mass lesion.

Pulmonary arteriography is reserved for those patients in whom embolectomy is being considered.

Chronic
1. 'Plump' hila with peripheral arterial pruning, i.e. the signs of pulmonary arterial hypertension.
2. ± multiple areas of linear atelectasis.

Further Reading
Chang C.H. (1967) Radiological considerations in pulmonary embolism. *Clin. Radiol.*, 18: 301–9.
Kerr I.H., Simon G. & Sutton G.C. (1971) The value of the plain radiograph in acute massive pulmonary embolism. *Br. J. Radiol.*, 44: 751–7.

Reiter's Syndrome

Sexually transmitted or following dysentery. Males predominate.

1. Urethritis ± cystitis ± prostatitis.
2. Circinate balanitis (30%).
3. Conjunctivitis (30%).
4. Keratoderma blennorrhagica.
5. Arthritis (radiological changes in 80% of cases)
   (a) Involvement of synovial and cartilaginous joints and entheses.
   (b) Asymmetrical involvement of the lower limbs — most commonly the knees, ankles, small joints of the feet and calcaneum. The spine and sacro-iliac joints are involved less frequently.
   (c) Soft-tissue swelling.
   (d) Osteoporosis is a feature of the acute disease but not of recurrent or chronic disease.
   (e) Erosions which are initially periarticular and progress to involve the central portion of the articular surface.
   (f) Periosteal new bone.
   (g) New bone formation at ligament and tendon insertions.
   (h) Sacro-iliitis and spondylitis with paravertebral ossification.

Renal Osteodystrophy

Due to renal glomerular disease — mostly bilateral chronic pyelonephritis and chronic glomerulonephritis. It consists of osteomalacia or rickets + secondary hyperparathyroidism + osteosclerosis.

Children
1. Changes most marked in the skull, pelvis, scapulae, vertebrae and metaphyses of tubular bones.
2. Vertebral sclerosis may be confined to the upper and lower thirds of the bodies — 'rugger jersey' spine.
3. Soft-tissue calcification — less common than in adults.
4. Rickets — but the epiphyseal plate is less wide and the metaphysis is less cupped than in vitamin-D dependent rickets.
5. Secondary hyperparathyroidism — subperiosteal erosions and a 'rotting fence-post' appearance of the femoral necks.
6. Delayed skeletal maturation.

Adults
1. Hyperparathyroidism (q.v.).
2. Soft-tissue calcification is common, especially in arteries.
3. Osteosclerosis, including 'rugger jersey' spine.
4. Osteomalacia is mainly evident as Looser's zones.

Rheumatoid Arthritis

A multisystem collagen disorder in which joint disease is variably associated with other systemic manifestations.

1. A symmetrical arthritis of synovial joints, especially the metacarpophalangeal and proximal interphalangeal joints of the hands and feet, wrists, knees, ankles, elbows, glenohumeral and acromioclavicular joints and hips. The synovial articulations of the axial skeleton may also be affected, especially the apophyseal and atlantoaxial joints of the cervical spine. Less commonly the sacroiliac and temperomandibular joints are involved.
2. Cartilaginous joints, e.g. discovertebral junctions outside the cervical spine, symphysis pubis and manubriosternal joints, and entheses are less frequently and less severely involved (c.f. seronegative spondyloarthropathies).
3. The sequence of pathological/radiological changes at synovial joints is
   (a) Synovial inflammation and effusion → soft-tissue swelling and widened joint space.
   (b) Hyperaemia and disuse → juxta-articular osteoporosis; later generalized.
   (c) Destruction of cartilage by pannus → joint-space narrowing.
   (d) Pannus destruction of unprotected bone at the insertion of the joint capsule → periarticular erosions.
   (e) Pannus destruction of subchondral bone → widespread erosions and subchondral cysts.
   (f) Capsular and ligamentous laxity → subluxation, dislocation and deformity.
   (g) Fibrous and bony ankylosis.
4. Periosteal reaction — uncommon.
5. Secondary degenerative arthritis in the major weight-bearing joints.

Complications
  1. Joint complications
     (a) Deformity and subluxation.
     (b) Pyogenic arthritis.
     (c) Tendon rupture.
     (d) Baker's cyst — which may rupture.
     (e) Cord or root compression due to cervical subluxation.
     (f) Hoarseness — due to involvement of the cricoarytenoid joints.
  2. Subcutaneous nodules.
  3. Anaemia.
  4. Pulmonary complications
     (a) Pleural effusion.
     (b) Rheumatoid nodules.
     (c) Fibrosing alveolitis.
     (d) Caplan's syndrome.
  5. Cardiac complications
     (a) Pericarditis ± effusion.
  6. Ocular complications
     (a) Episcleritis.
     (b) Uveitis.
     (c) Sjögren's syndrome.
  7. Arteritis
     (a) Raynaud's phenomenon.
     (b) Leg ulcers.
     (c) Visceral ischaemia.
  8. Felty's syndrome (splenomegaly, leucopenia and rheumatoid arthritis).
  9. Peripheral and autonomic neuropathy.
 10. Amyloidosis.
 11. Complications of therapy.

Rickets

Increased uncalcified osteoid in the immature skeleton.

Changes at the Growth Plate and Cortex

1. Widened growth plate (a).
2. Fraying, splaying and cupping of the metaphysis, which is of reduced density (b).
3. Thin bony spur extending from the metaphysis to surround the uncalcified growth plate (c).
4. Indistinct cortex because of uncalcified subperiosteal osteoid (d).
5. Rickety rosary — cupping of the anterior ends of the ribs and, on palpation, abnormally large costochondral junctions.
6. Looser's zones · uncommon in children.

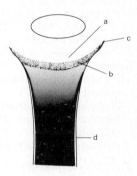

Changes Due to Bone Softening (Deformities)

1. Bowing of long bones.
2. Triradiate pelvis.
3. Harrison's sulcus — indrawing of the lower part of the chest wall because of soft ribs.
4. Scoliosis.
5. Biconcave vertebral bodies.
6. Basilar invagination.
7. Craniotabes — flattening of the occiput and accumulating osteoid in the frontal and parietal regions.

General Changes

1. Retarded bone maturation and growth.
2. Decreased bone density — uncommon.

Sarcoidosis

A multisystem granulomatous disorder of unknown aetiology.
Commonest presentations are:

erythema nodosum	30%
routine chest X-ray	25%
respiratory symptoms	20%
ocular symptoms	8%
other skin lesions	5%.

Intrathoracic Sarcoidosis (in 90%)
The chest X-ray at presentation may be:

normal	8%
bilateral hilar lymphadenopathy (BHL)	50%
bilateral hilar lymphadenopathy + pulmonary infiltrate	30%
pulmonary infiltrate ± fibrosis	12%.

1. Lymphadenopathy — bilateral hilar ± uni- or bilateral paratracheal lymphadenopathy. Anterior mediastinal lymph nodes are also involved in 16%. Unilateral hilar lymphadenopathy in 1–5%. 'Eggshell' calcification occurs in 1–5% and takes about 6 years to develop.
2. Parenchymal shadowing includes
   (a) Micronodular shadows < 2 mm ⎱ predominantly
   (b) Larger shadows < 5 mm, ill defined, ⎰ mid mimicking consolidation or oedema ⎰ zones.
   (c) Large nodules, 1–4 cm, ill defined, multiple, bilateral and in any zone.
   (d) Coarse fibrosis — typically in the mid and upper zones.
3. Pleural involvement in 5–7%. Effusion in 2%.
4. Pneumothorax — secondary to chronic lung fibrosis.
5. Bronchostenosis in 1–2% — extrinsic compression or endobronchial granuloma.

Skin Sarcoidosis
1. Erythema nodosum — almost always in association with bilateral hilar lymphadenopathy.
2. Lupus pernio, plaques, subcutaneous nodules and scar infiltration.

Ocular Sarcoidosis
1. Most commonly manifests as acute uveitis + bilateral hilar lymphadenopathy + erythema nodosum.

Hepatic and Gastrointestinal Sarcoidosis
1. Hepatic granulomas in 66%, but symptomatic hepatobiliary disease is rare.
2. Gastric and peritoneal granulomas occur but are asymptomatic.

Neurologic Sarcoidosis
1. Neuropathies — especially bilateral lower motor neurone VII nerve palsies.
2. Cerebral sarcoidosis is evident in 14% of autopsies of patients dying of sarcoidosis, but in only 1–5% clinically. Most commonly it produces nodular granulomatous masses in the basal meninges or adhesive meningitis, which result in cranial nerve palsies and/or hydrocephalus. Granulomas in the brain parenchyma present as space-occupying lesions. (On CT scanning they have a high attenuation, are homogeneously enhancing and peripherally situated.)

Joint Sarcoidosis
1. A transient, symmetrical arthropathy involving knees, ankles and, less commonly, the wrists and interphalangeal joints.

Bone Sarcoidosis
1. In 3% of patients and most frequently associated with skin lesions.
2. Hands and feet are most commonly affected
    (a) Enlarged nutrient foramina in phalanges and, occasionally, metacarpals and metatarsals.
    (b) Coarse trabeculation, eventually assuming a lacework, reticulated pattern. Initially metaphyseal and eventually affecting the entire bone.
    (c) Larger, well-defined lucencies.
    (d) Resorption of distal phalanges.
    (e) Terminal phalangeal sclerosis.
    (f) Periarticular calcification.
    (g) Subperiosteal bone resorption — simulating hyperparathyroidism.
    (h) Periosteal reaction.
    (i) Soft-tissue swelling — dactylitis.

3. In the remainder of the skeleton
   (a) Well-defined lucencies with a sclerotic margin.
   (b) Paraspinal masses with an extradural block at myelography.
   (c) Destructive lesions of the nasal and jaw bones.

Sarcoidosis Elsewhere
1. Peripheral lymphadenopathy in 15%.
2. Hypercalcaemia (10%) and hypercalciuria (60%).
3. Splenomegaly in 6%.
4. Uveoparotid fever (uveitis, cranial nerve palsy, fever and parotitis).

Further Reading
Freundlich I.M., Libshitz H.I., Glassman L.M. & Israel H.L., (1970) Sarcoidosis: typical and atypical thoracic manifestations and complications. *Clin. Radiol.*, 21: 376–83.
Kendall B.E. (1978). Radiological findings in neurosarcoidosis. *Br. J. Radiol.*, 51: 81–92.

Scleroderma (Progressive Systemic Sclerosis)

A multisystem connective tissue disorder, the course of which varies from acute and fulminating to mild and chronic.

Soft Tissues
1. Raynaud's phenomenon (60%).
2. Skin thickening — initially of the fingers (and less often the toes) and of the mouth; progresses to shiny taut skin.
3. Subcutaneous calcification — especially in the fingertips and over bony prominences.
4. Myopathy or myositis.

Joints
1. Eventually 50% of patients have articular involvement. Fingers, wrists and ankles are commonly affected.
2. Terminal phalangeal resorption is associated with soft-tissue atrophy.
3. Erosions at the distal interphalangeal, 1st carpometacarpal, metacarpophalangeal and metatarsophalangeal joints.

Mandible
1. Thickening of the periodontal membrane ± loss of the lamina dura.

Ribs
1. Symmetrical erosions on the superior surfaces which predominate along the posterior aspects of the 3rd–6th ribs.

Respiratory System
1. Lung involvement in 10–25%.
2. Aspiration pneumonitis secondary to gastro-oesophageal reflux.
3. Interstitial lung disease and fibrosis, more marked in the lower zones.

Gastrointestinal System

1. Oesophageal abnormalities (50%) — dilatation, atonicity, poor or absent peristalsis and free gastro-oesophageal reflux through a widely open gastro-oesophageal junction.
2. Small bowel (75%) — dilated, atonic, thickened mucosal folds and pseudosacculation.
3. Colon (75%) — atonic with pseudosacculations on the antimesenteric border.

Heart

1. Cardiomegaly (30%) — due to myocardial ± pericardial involvement. ± pericardial effusion.
2. Cor pulmonale may develop secondary to the interstitial lung disease.

Scurvy

The result of vitamin-C deficiency.

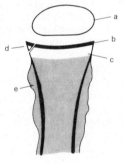

1. Onset at 6 months – 2 years. Rare in adults.
2. Earliest signs are seen at the knees.
3. Osteoporosis (usually the only sign seen in adults).
4. Loss of epiphyseal density with a pencil-thin cortex (Wimberger's sign) (a).
5. Dense zone of provisional calcification — due to excessive calcification of osteoid (b).
6. Metaphyseal lucency (Trümmerfeld zone) (c).
7. Metaphyseal corner fractures through the weakened lucent metaphysis (Pelkan spurs) resulting in cupping of the metaphysis (d).
8. Periosteal reaction due to subperiosteal haematoma (e).

Sickle-cell Anaemia

Skeletal
1. Marrow hyperplasia produces widening of medullary cavities, decreased bone density, coarsening of the trabecular pattern, and cortical thinning and expansion. The changes are most marked in the axial skeleton.
   (a) Skull — coarse granular osteoporosis with widening of the diploe which spares the occiput below the internal occipital protuberance. 'Hair-on-end' appearance (5%). Focal lucencies (but probably due to infarcts).
   (b) Spine — osteoporosis, exaggerated vertical trabeculae and biconcave vertebral bodies (but see also 2(c) below).
2. Vascular occlusion due to sickling results in osteonecrosis.
   (a) Sickle-cell dactylitis (hand–foot syndrome) — in children aged 6 months – 2 years. Symmetrical soft-tissue swelling, patchy lucency and sclerosis of the shafts of metacarpals, metatarsals and phalanges, and periosteal reaction.
   (b) Long bones — diaphyseal or epiphyseal infarcts. The femoral head is affected in 12% of patients (60% in sickle/haemoglobin C (SC) disease).
   (c) Spine — square-shaped compression infarcts of the vertebral end-plates are virtually diagnostic.
3. Growth disturbances — retarded growth, delayed closure of epiphyses and tibiotalar slant.
4. Fractures.
5. Osteomyelitis and pyogenic arthritis — due to salmonellae in over 50% of cases.

Extraskeletal
1. Extramedullary haemopoiesis — but more common in thalassaemia.
2. Cholelithiasis.
3. Splenic infarction.
4. Cardiomegaly and congestive cardiac failure — because of anaemia.
5. Renal papillary necrosis.

Silicosis

Occurs in miners, quarry workers, masons, pottery workers, sand blasters, foundry workers and boiler scalers. The duration and degree of exposure determine the time of onset of disease
(a) Chronic silicosis — disease after 20–40 years of exposure.
(b) Accelerated silicosis — disease after 5–15 years of exposure.
(c) Acute silicoproteinosis — heavy exposure over a short period of time (several months – 5 years), e.g. in sand blasters.

Simple
1. Nodular shadows, pin-point to pea-sized, which are first seen around the right hilum but later are disseminated throughout both lungs with relative sparing of the extreme bases and apices. Exceptionally, they may be restricted to the upper zones.
2. Inhalation of pure silica produces very sharp, dense nodules. Mixed dusts are less well defined and of lower density. Density increases with the size of the nodule. Goldminers have very dense nodular shadows.
3. Nodules may calcify, especially in goldminers.
4. Minor hilar lymph-node enlargement, but only obvious when calcification occurs (in 5%). Anterior and posterior mediastinal lymph nodes may also enlarge.
5. Kerley A and B lines — more pronounced with mixed dusts.
6. Silicoproteinosis presents as diffuse alveolar disease.

Complicated, i.e. Progressive Massive Fibrosis (PMF)
1. Superimposed on the changes of simple silicosis.
2. The rapid development of massive, ill-defined, dense, oval or round shadows. Usually bilateral and fairly symmetrical in the upper two-thirds of the lungs.
3. They begin peripherally and increase in size and density as they move towards the hilum, leaving emphysematous lung at the periphery.
4. May cavitate or calcify.

Complications
1. Infections — chronic bronchitis and tuberculosis.
2. Pneumothorax — but usually limited by thickened pleura.
3. Cor pulmonale — a common cause of death.
4. Caplan's syndrome — in patients with rheumatoid disease. Well-defined, peripheral nodules 0.5–5 cm in diameter. Calcification and cavitation may occur.

Simple Bone Cyst

1. Age — 5–15 years.
2. Sites — proximal humerus and femur (75% of cases) and apophysis of the greater trochanter.
3. Appearances
   (a) Metaphyseal, extending to the epiphyseal plate. It migrates away from the metaphysis with time.
   (b) Well-defined lucency with a thin sclerotic rim.
   (c) Usually central.
   (d) Thinned cortex with slight expansion (never more than the width of the epiphyseal plate).
   (e) Thin internal septa.

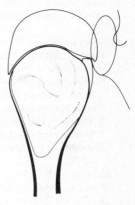

Steroids

See 'Cushing's syndrome'.

Systemic Lupus Erythematosus

Musculoskeletal

1. Polyarthritis — bilateral and symmetrical, involving the small joints of the hand, knee, wrist and shoulder. Soft-tissue swelling and periarticular osteoporosis of the proximal interphalangeal and metacarpophalangeal joints simulate rheumatoid arthritis, but periarticular erosions are not a usual feature.
2. Easily correctable deformities of the hand which cause little functional disability.
3. Osteonecrosis — most frequently of the femoral head.
4. Terminal phalangeal sclerosis and resorption.

Cardiorespiratory

1. Pleural effusion (60%), which is often recurrent. Often accompanied by a pleurisy resulting in elevation of a hemidiaphragm and plate atelectasis at the base.
2. Uraemic pulmonary oedema.
3. Acute lupus pneumonitis.
4. Diffuse interstitial disease — uncommon.
5. Cardiomegaly — due to pericarditis with effusion, myocardial disease or fluid overload in renal failure.

Abdomen

1. Hepatosplenomegaly.
2. Renal disease eventually results in small, smooth, non-functioning kidneys.

Thalassaemia

Skeletal
1. Marrow hyperplasia is more pronounced than in sickle-cell anaemia (q.v.). The changes in thalassaemia major are more severe than in thalassaemia minor. Initially both axial and appendicular skeleton are affected but as marrow regresses from the appendicular skeleton at puberty the changes in the latter diminish.
   (a) Skull — granular osteoporosis, widening of the diploe, thinning of the outer table and 'hair-on-end' appearance. Involvement of the facial bones produces obliteration of the paranasal sinuses, hypertelorism and malocclusion of the teeth. These changes are rarely a feature of other haemoglobinopathies and are important differentiating signs.
   (b) Spine — osteoporosis, exaggerated vertical trabeculae and fish-shaped vertebrae.
   (c) Ribs, clavicles and tubular bones of the hands and feet show the typical changes of marrow hyperplasia (see Sickle-cell anaemia).
2. Growth disturbances.
3. Fractures.

Extraskeletal
1. Extramedullary haemopoiesis — including hepatosplenomegaly.
2. Cardiomegaly.

Tuberous Sclerosis

Autosomal dominant. 25–50% are fresh mutations.
Mental retardation in 60%. 30% die in the first 5 years; 75% are dead by 20 years.

Central Nervous System
1. Cortical and/or subependymal periventricular nodules. Calcification in 50–80%, but not visible until after infancy.
2. Ventricular dilatation, with or without obstruction.
3. Gliomas in 6%.
4. Retinal tumours (phakomas) in 50%; 60% are bilateral.

Skin
1. Adenoma sebaceum, subungual fibromas, shagreen patches and cafe-au-lait spots.

Kidneys
1. Hamartomas (angiomyolipomas) in 50–80%. Single or multiple, uni- or bilateral. (N.B. approx. 50% of patients with an angiomyolipoma have no other evidence of tuberous sclerosis.)

Skeleton
1. Calvarium, spine and pelvis — sclerotic islands in 40–50%.
2. Hands and feet — cystic defects and periosteal new bone, especially in the phalanges. The changes are more marked in the hands.

Lungs
1. Interstitial lung disease progressing to 'honeycomb lung' in 5%. Never before 20 years. A frequent cause of death.

Heart
1. Cardiac rhabdomyomas. The chest X-ray is normal or shows non-specific cardiac enlargement.

Further Reading
Medley B.E., McLeod R.A. & Wayne Houser O. (1976) Tuberous sclerosis. *Semin. Roentgenol.*, 11: 35–54.

Turner's Syndrome

Females with XO chromosome pattern.

1. Small stature with retarded bone maturation.
2. Mental retardation in 10%.
3. Osteoporosis.

Chest
1. Cardiovascular abnormalities — present in 20%, and 70% are coarctation.
2. Broad chest; mild pectus excavatum; widely spaced nipples.

Abdomen
1. Ovarian dysgenesis.
2. Renal anomalies — 'horseshoe kidney' and bifid renal pelvis are the most common.

Axial Skeleton
1. Scoliosis and kyphosis.
2. Hypoplasia of the cervical spine.

Appendicular Skeleton
1. Cubitus valgus in 70%.
2. Short 4th metacarpal and/or metatarsal in 50%, ± short 3rd and 5th metacarpals.
3. Madelung's deformity.
4. Enlargement of the medial tibial plateau ± small exostosis inferiorly.
5. Pes cavus.
6. Transient congenital oedema of the dorsum of the feet.

Ulcerative Colitis

1. Diseased colon is affected in continuity with symmetrical involvement of the wall.
2. Rectum involved in 95%. The rectum may appear normal if steroid enemas have been administered.
3. Granular mucosa and mucosal ulcers.
4. 'Thumbprinting' due mucosal oedema.
5. Blunting of haustral folds progresses to a narrowed, shortened and tubular colon if the disease becomes chronic.
6. Widening of the retrorectal space.
7. Inflammatory pseudopolyps due to regenerating mucosa. Found in 10–20% of ulcerative colitics and usually following a previous severe attack. Filiform polyps occur in quiescent phase.
8. Patulous ileocaecal valve with reflux ileitis (dilated terminal ileum).

Complications
1. Toxic megacolon — in 7–10%.
2. Strictures — much less common than in Crohn's disease and must be differentiated from carcinoma.
3. Carcinoma of the colon — 20–30× increased incidence if extensive colitis has been present for more than 10 years.
4. Associated conditions
   (a) Erythema nodosum, aphthous ulceration and pyoderma gangrenosum.
   (b) Arthritis — similar to Crohn's disease (q.v.).
   (c) Cirrhosis.
   (d) Chronic active hepatitis.
   (e) Pericholangitis.
   (f) Sclerosing cholangitis.
   (g) Bile duct carcinoma.
   (h) Oxalate urinary calculi.

Index

Part 1 is indexed by sections
Part 2 is indexed by page numbers
References in **bold** type are to principal sections

pneumoconioses (*cont.*)
   septal (Kerley B) lines 4.18
pneumocystis carinii pneumonia 4.14
pneumomediastinum **4.37**
   pneumoperitoneum 6.2
   post-tracheal/bronchial laceration/
      fracture 4.43
pneumonia
   alveolar opacities
      localized **4.15**
      widespread **4.14**
      + enlarged hilum **4.10**
   increased density of hemithorax
      4.7
   neonatal respiratory distress 4.44
   pneumothorax 4.36
   pulmonary nodule 4.24
   pulmonary opacities 4.23
      with air bronchogram 4.27
   slowly resolving/recurrent **4.9**
pneumonia, aspiration
   increased density of hemithorax
      4.7
   pulmonary opacities 4.23
pneumonia, lobar **4.11**
pneumonia, perihilar 4.29
pneumonia, staphylococcal 4.8
pneumonia, viral
   alveolar opacities 4.14
   pneumonia + enlarged hilum 4.10
pneumonitis, aspiration: post-chest
    trauma 4.43
pneumonitis, chemical 4.20
pneumonitis, diffuse
   drug-induced 4.46
      + systemic lupus erythematosus
      4.46
pneumonitis, radiation 4.27
pneumoperitoneum 6.1, **6.2**
   bilateral elevated hemidiaphragms
      4.39
   idiopathic 6.2
   iatrogenic 6.2
   pneumothorax 4.36
pneumothorax **4.36**
   'honeycomb lung' 4.36
   hypertransradiant hemithorax,
      unilateral 4.4
   pneumoperitoneum 6.2
   post-chest trauma 4.43
   spontaneous 4.36
poisons: pulmonary oedema 4.16
Poland's syndrome 4.4
poliomyelitis
   hypertransradiant hemithorax 4.4
   rib notching 1.42
   scoliosis 2.1
polyarteritis nodosa
   aphthoid ulcers 6.41
   kidneys, large smooth 8.10

pulmonary arteries enlarged 5.15
renal induced hypertension 8.18
right ventricle enlarged 5.4
polycalycosis 8.21
polycystic disease
   abdominal mass in neonate 6.5
   adult 8.9, 8.13, **323**
   hepatomegaly 7.5
   infantile 8.13, **322**
   kidneys, large smooth 8.10
   nephrogram 8.16
   renal induced hypertension 8.18
   respiratory distress, neonatal 4.44
polycythaemia rubra vera
   avascular necrosis 1.36
   hepatomegaly 7.5
polyvinyl chloride tank cleaners:
    phalangeal resorption 1.44
porencephalic cyst: CT 11.28, 11.29
portal hypertension: splenomegaly
    7.7
portal vein
   gas in 6.1, **7.4**
   preduodenal: intestinal obstruction
      in neonate 6.7
post-cricoid carcinoma 10.15
posterior cranial fossa neoplasms **11.27**
posterior urethral valves:
    hydronephrosis 6.5
post-lymphogram pulmonary
    opacities 4.21
post-pneumonectomy: increased
    density of hemithorax 4.7
potassium tablets enteric-coated,
    small bowel strictures 6.28
Pott's procedure: pulmonary oedema
    4.17
pregnancy
   avascular necrosis 1.36
   azygos vein enlarged 5.14
   bilateral elevated hemidiaphragm
      4.39
   symphysis pubis widening 3.14
presbyoesophagus 6.15
prevertebral cervical region soft-
    tissue mass **10.15**
primary acro-osteolysis 11.13
progeria
   osteoporosis 1.26
   rib notching 1.42
progressive diaphyseal dysplasia
    (Engelmann's disease) 1.5
progressive systemic sclerosis *see*
    scleroderma
prolactinoma 11.19
   CT 11.28, 11.29
prostate carcinoma: bone metastases
    1.13
   see also entries under
     osteoblastic metastases